THE LITTLE BLACK DRESS DIET

Michael van Straten is the UK's best known practitioner of complementary medicine. As well as two very busy practices in London and Buckinghamshire, he has become the voice of natural therapy throughout the country.

His radio show 'Bodytalk' on London's LBC has been running for 25 years and he's also a regular guest on radio programmes throughout the country. He's appeared on most of the TV chat shows and has been a regular on breakfast TV and many other food and health programmes, including the controversial Central Weekend Live. Michael is often to be seen on the Carlton Taste Channel, for whom he recently made a series on growing and cooking with herbs.

A prolific writer with more than 20 books already published, including the bestselling *Super Juice and The Good Sleep Guide,* Michael is in constant demand as a lecturer at public meetings and conferences here and abroad, and his books have been translated into many languages including Japanese.

His favourite hobby is baking bread and making jams and pickles from the organic produce his wife Sally grows in their garden.

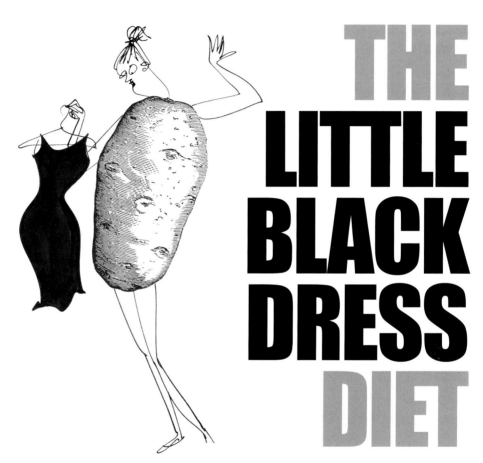

THE LITTLE BLACK DRESS DIET

MICHAEL VAN STRATEN

with recipes by sally pearce and michael van straten

KYLE CATHIE LIMITED

First published in Great Britain in 2001 by
Kyle Cathie Limited
122 Arlington Road
London NW1 7HP
general.enquiries@kyle-cathie.com
www.kylecathie.com

Reprinted 2001, 2002, 2003

ISBN 1 85626 431 9

The Publishers would like to thank the Kobal Collection for
the photographs that appear in this book.

Editor: Kyle Cathie
Designer: Geoff Hayes
Production: Lorraine Baird & Sha Huxtable
Repro: Colourpath Limited London
Printed by Colorcraft Limited Hong Kong

FOR SALLY

I've spent almost 40 years helping other people to lose
weight but nothing brings the problems home like going
through it yourself. After an accident I needed spinal
surgery but I had lose two stone quickly. Forced to practise
what I had preached for so long and to carry on losing
weight during a painful period of recuperation, I know how
hard it is.

Without the tireless support of my wife **Sally** this book
would never have been written. While I laid on my back
dictating, **Sally** would say in more ways than one she was
nurse, chauffeur and recipe creator. And that's going to cost
me a very expensive **Little Black Dress**.

I would also like to dedicate it to the wonderful nursing
staff on the neurosurgery ward at The Wellington Hospital,
London, especially Sister Suzie. Without her 3a.m. cups of
Horlicks and constant support, life would have been very
difficult.

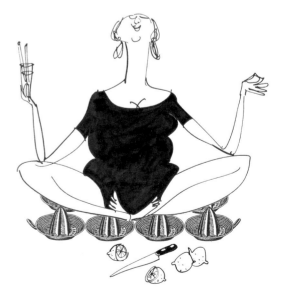

courgette is zucchini squash

CONTENTS

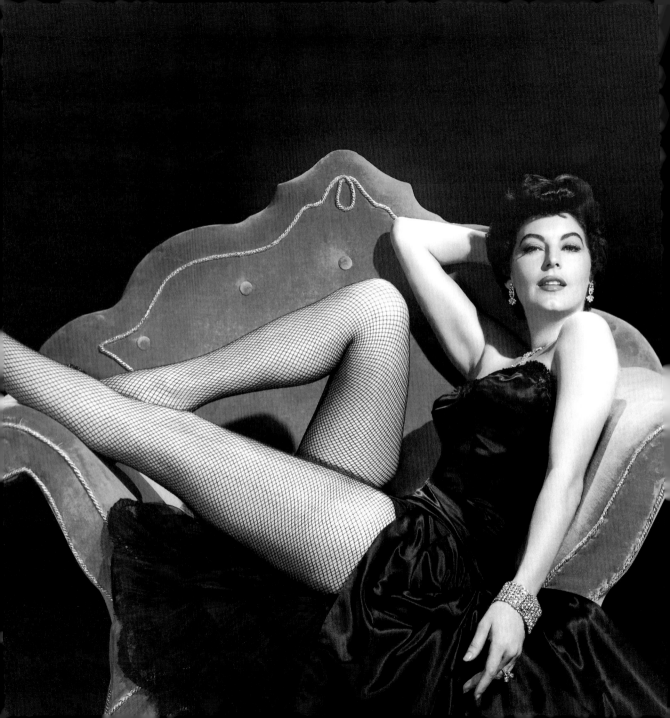

INTRODUCTION

We've all been there – a hot date, dinner with the boss, a smart Christmas cocktail party – and you suddenly realise you're mysteriously a size larger than you were when you bought that expensive little black number. Or the chaps discover that the cummerbund won't quite cover the flesh-revealing gap between the popping buttons on their dress shirt. Disaster!

The temptation, then, is to throw out the entire contents of the fridge and live on a diet of water and carrots. As a naturopath, however, I can tell you that crash diets don't work. They're not healthy and, on less than 1,000 calories a day, it's impossible to get all the nutrients and sustain the energy you need to lead a normal life. In any case, from the minute you stop dieting, you put on all the weight you've lost, plus some. That said, however, there are times when people really need to lose weight quickly – if, for example, they have to go into hospital for an operation or their excess weight is putting severe strain on already-damaged muscles, joints or tendons. Yes, and for that special occasion. That's when you need the Little Black Dress Diet – or, of course, the Black Tie Diet for the men.

We live in a crazy world, a world in which conflicting messages and commercial interests all conspire against us: the health messages that warn of the dangers of being overweight; the advertising messages that urge us to buy high-fat, high-sugar and high-salt foods; the fashion messages which show size 10 models in the glamorous clothes you'd all love to wear; the celebrity icons which every teenager

wants to emulate, including their personal trainers, life coaches and diet gurus. And wherever you look, advertisers use these images of glamorous thinness to sell everything.

The food, drink, snack, crisp and nut manufacturers spend billions of pounds persuading us to buy their predominantly unhealthy products, but when did you last see an advert for a cabbage, a carrot or a cauliflower? Health education has always been a Cinderella, so it's up to you to grasp the nettle – and eat it, too, as you'll see in later recipes – if you want to get into that little black dress or DJ.

As well as The Little Black Dress diet, you'll find a whole selection of other diet plans to suit different situations. You can beat the bloat, enjoy a veggie weight-loss feast, there's a special Black Tie diet for the guys and even a desperation diet when the few extra pounds become a major crisis. As well as all you need to know about good nutrition, you can discover the real way to find out whether you have any genuine food allergies or intolerances before you give up wheat, gluten and dairy products on the say-so of some untrained person with a totally bogus machine.

And here's the best news of all: you don't need to know how many calories there are in the recipes and there is absolutely no need to weigh every ingredient or portion to the nearest micro-gram. Just remember that eating is one of life's great pleasures – and to forego them all just for the sake of a few grams here or there makes a mockery of the whole concept of healthy living. What matters is what you do most of the time and the occasional 'lapse' of a bar of chocolate, a real ice-cream or a deliciously creamy pud doesn't matter. After all, holistic health means taking care of mind, body and soul and a little of what you fancy always takes care of the soul.

Ava Gardner, 1952

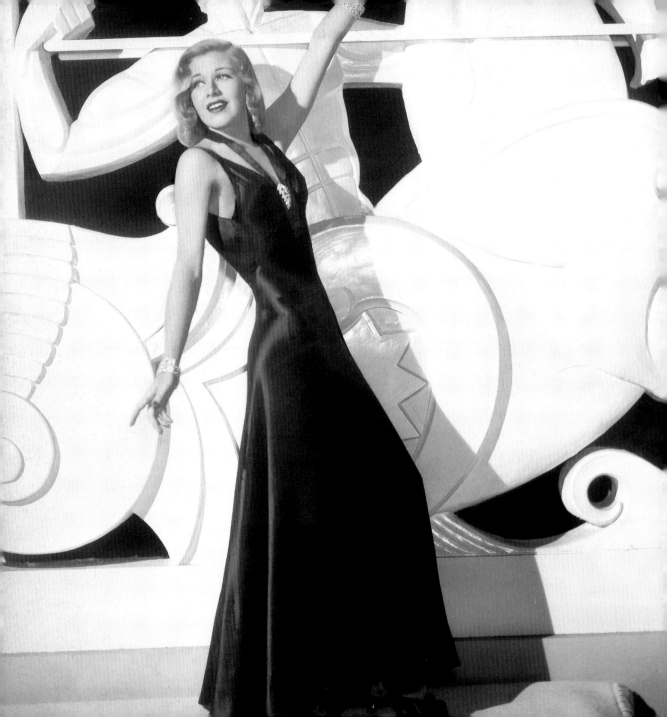

THE LITTLE BLACK DRESS DIET

Don't panic, your worries are over. If you've got a wardrobe full of little black dresses, a two-week deadline to a really important occasion and you can't get into any of them, here's the solution.

This is a 10-day regime which I've used for my patients for many years with great success. It's normally reserved for those medical emergencies like impending surgery or a sudden rise in blood pressure, but I suppose you could stretch the point and call the little black dress disaster an emergency. After all, your career or love life – possibly even both – could depend on it.

Follow this plan and you really can lose 4-5kg/10lb in 10 days with this healthy eating regime, which is loosely based on the principles of food combining (page 48). The first three days are fairly drastic, but after that you shouldn't feel hungry or tired and you will enjoy real food. Ideally, start the diet at a weekend or when you don't have to work for two or three days. The basic principle is that you don't mix starch and protein in the same meal. People talk a lot of pseudo-scientific claptrap about food combining and the

truth is, I've no idea why it works, but I can promise you that it does – although there's absolutely no medical reason why it should.

Any eating plan which makes you follow a regime and eat regular meals will help you lose weight. The Little Black Dress Diet encourages you to eat real food in the sort of quantities that will provide most people with more calories than they normally eat, but they're healthy calories. And that's all you need to know to achieve your goal.

All the recipes in this book are interchangeable during the 10 days of this diet, just make sure that you substitute like for like – salad for salad, fish for fish etc. As well as the food, make sure that you take 3 teaspoons a day of the Swiss herbal tonic Bio-Strath Elixir to boost your natural immunity, 1 Genesis vitamin and mineral pill as extra health insurance and that you have at least 1 litre/2 1/2 pints of water with a measure of the natural detox herbal remedy Pure Plan every day in addition to your normal drinks. For this 10 days, keep off the alcohol if you really want to lose the weight.

Ginger Rogers in Top Hat, *1935*

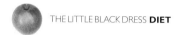

DAY 1

Breakfast: a large melon.

Light meal or snack: vegetable soup or carrot and celery juice.
Raw Veg and Brown Rice Salad (page 91).

Main meal: mixed salad.
Any cooked green vegetables with a can of your favourite beans (not baked, and well-rinsed) and 1 teaspoon olive oil.

DAY 2

Breakfast: freshly juiced apple and carrot or fresh orange.

Light meal or snack: the rest of yesterday's soup.
Salad.
Baked sweet potatoes.

Main meal: salad, cooked green vegetables.
Cooked cauliflower sprinkled with grated cheese and browned under the grill.

DAY 3

Breakfast: a cup of hot water mixed with soya milk and
2 tablespoons molasses.
2 slices of wholewheat bread and butter.

Light meal or snack: large selection of fruit with raisins and dates.

Main meal: salad. Cooked green vegetables. Whole-wheat pasta and tomato sauce.

DAY 4

Breakfast: half a grapefruit.
Apple.
Natural yoghurt with a little honey and chopped nuts.

Light meal or snack: baked potato with butter or 1 tablespoon sour cream and chopped fresh herbs.
Three-Colour Coleslaw (page 87).
A ripe sweet pear.

Main meal: Vegetable and Cheese Casserole (page 75) served with steamed broccoli.
Orange.

DAY 5

Breakfast: porridge made with water and 1 tablespoon single cream.
1 slice wholewheat bread or toast with a little butter.

Light meal or snack: Winter Salad (page 87).
Stewed apple.

Main meal: Green Goodness (page 100).
Grilled Spiced Chicken (page 76) served with steamed leeks and carrots.

DAY 6

Breakfast: Scrambled Eggs with Mushrooms (page 61).
Orange juice.

Light meal or snack: Curried Pumpkin Soup (page 101).
Wholewheat roll and butter.
Watercress, Avocado and Celery Salad (page 90).

Main meal: Mighty Hummus (page 103) with celery, carrot and
fennel sticks.
Stuffed Grilled Trout (page 76).
Steamed green cabbage.

DAY 7

Breakfast: grapefruit juice.
Stewed apples sprinkled with flaked almonds.
Natural yoghurt.

Light meal or snack: Mushroom Risotto (page 79).
A tossed green salad.
A ripe sweet pear.

Main meal: Easy Lamb Stir-Fry (page 77).
Sticks of celery and an apple.

DAY 8

Breakfast: homemade Real Swiss Muesli (page 60) with a sliced
banana and a little single cream.

Light meal or snack: large baked potato with baked beans.
Chicory and Watercress Salad (page 90).

Main meal: Fruity, Spicy Carrot Soup (page100).
Cod with Yoghurt Crust (page 78) served with a mixed salad.

DAY 9

Breakfast: Breakfast Compôte (page 63) with 1 tablespoon
Greek yoghurt.

Light meal or snack: hot wholemeal pitta filled with Mighty
Hummus (page 103), spring onions, tomato and lettuce.
Bunch of grapes.
Banana.

Main meal: half a grapefruit. Avocado Salmon (page 69). Cauliflower
purée. Tossed green salad.

DAY 10

Breakfast: 2 rashers lean grilled bacon with 1 scrambled egg,
mushrooms and large grilled tomato.

Light meal or snack: Winter Salad (see page 87).
Apple.

Main meal: small Prawn and Avocado Salad (page 91).
Aromatic Lamb (page 73) with a purée of turnips and carrots.
Celery sticks and selection of cheese.

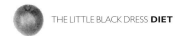

PACKED LUNCHES

Planning packed lunches that are either starch or protein is certainly trickier than making up a few sandwiches with cheese, salami or cold chicken, adding a carton of yoghurt, perhaps, and an apple. But these suggestions for a working week of both starch- and protein-packed lunches are simple substitutes for the midday meals in the diet plan.

If you're cooking rice for dinner, make extra, add dressing while it's still hot and pack it for lunch the next morning, adding pieces of cucumber, tomato, black olives, cress, spring onions or whatever salad stuff you have. Make extra quantities of comforting thick vegetable soups in the evening, save some for the next day's lunch and take in a thermos.

A WEEK OF STARCH-PACKED LUNCHES

MONDAY: wholewheat pitta pocket stuffed with cucumber, tomato, watercress, black olives, lettuce and a dribble of olive oil. Raisins and nuts.

TUESDAY: wholewheat sandwiches with hard-boiled egg yolks mashed with low-fat mayonnaise, slices of cucumber and cress. 2 oatmeal biscuits. A banana.

WEDNESDAY: thermos of thick vegetable soup. A wholewheat roll or rye crackers with butter. Carrot salad with raisins and nuts. Banana.

THURSDAY: rice salad. Rye crispbread. A ripe sweet pear.

FRIDAY: sticks of carrot, celery, fennel, cucumber, sprigs of cauliflower with tzatsiki for dipping. Wholewheat roll with butter.

A WEEK OF PROTEIN-PACKED LUNCHES

MONDAY: natural cottage cheese. An apple. A hard-boiled egg. Chunks of carrot, celery, cucumber, fennel.

TUESDAY: cabbage, celery, apple and grated Gruyère cheese salad. Orange or grapes. 25g/1oz roasted almonds. Yoghurt.

WEDNESDAY: Crudités with guacamole. A carton of stewed apple with ginger with 2 tablespoons yoghurt stirred in. Assorted nuts.

THURSDAY: piece of cold roast chicken or slices of cold roast turkey breast. Apple, celery and peanut salad. Grapes.

FRIDAY: natural yoghurt. Sticks of celery. A piece of hard cheese. Apple. Dates

Congratulations. If you haven't cheated too much, you should have easily gone down a dress size if you needed to. Don't go out on the binge tomorrow and stuff yourself with chocolate, buns and booze. You've worked hard, so now you can reap the reward of your efforts. You could safely follow this diet for another 10 days if it's really vital and it's fine to repeat the whole process three or four times a year.

Don't forget that even a modest amount of extra exercise will allow you to eat a bit more, enjoy a couple of glasses of wine a day – and the occasional indulgence – without putting back that lost weight. Why not buy a skipping rope – 10 minutes of skipping a day equals a couple of cream cakes?

There's nothing more disheartening than working really hard just so that you can get into that little black dress for a special occasion and a month later finding that you're back to square one and the whole process has to start again. If this has been the story of your life, now's the time to turn over a new leaf. **Now's the time to make permanent changes that are much simpler than you think. Now's the time to put all those years of one diet after another behind you. Now's the time to turn to the next chapter for the sane life-long plan to maintain a healthy weight.**

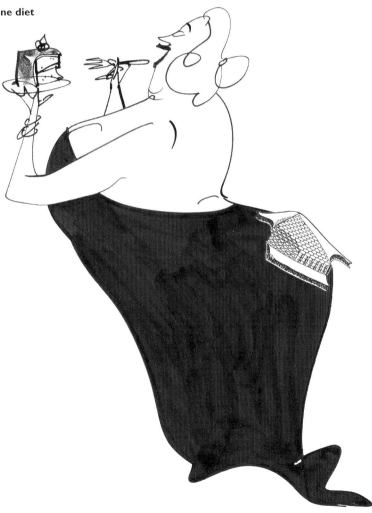

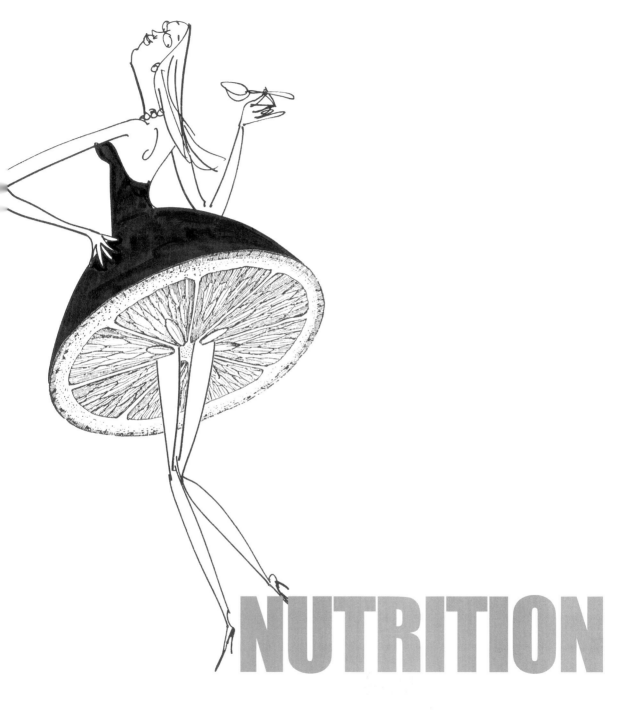

NUTRITION

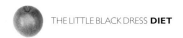

Eating well and maintaining the weight you want doesn't involve a magical mystery tour of supermarkets, health food stores or strange shops. All you need is a little basic understanding of what your body requires and how to translate those requirements into delicious meals.

Let's be clear right at the start that being thin isn't a guarantee of good health, and being modestly overweight is certainly not a recipe for disaster. It's worth noting that your life expectancy will be statistically shorter if you're 10 per cent underweight than it will be if you're 10 per cent overweight.

The risk of osteoporosis, the dreadful brittle bone disease which cripples many thousands of women each year, is far greater in those who are underweight. Thin elderly women are much more likely to fracture a hip after a simple fall than their more cuddly counterparts.

Of course, being obese is a very different matter, as you'll see. But being one dress size larger in your 30s than in your teens doesn't mean obesity, and being slim is no protection against high blood pressure, strokes and heart disease – particularly if you smoke, have raised cholesterol, eat lots of salt and don't take any exercise.

Here are some simple guidelines that will help you achieve your goals without deprivation or depression. Eat lots of

• Good carbohydrates, like wholemeal bread, brown rice, potatoes, root vegetables, beans and pasta, all for their high energy, slow release calories and zero fat content.

• Fresh fruits, vegetables and salads to provide vitamins, minerals and fibre.

• Fish, poultry without skin.

Cut down on

• All visible fats – if you see it don't eat it.

• Alcohol – have just one unit a day.

• Your consumption of all processed meat products.

• Avoid sugar, full-fat dairy products, all high-fat, high-sugar biscuits, cakes, desserts, sweets and chocolates.

Of all the nutritional disorders that affect the total population, obesity is the most common in affluent society. It's a major disease of civilisation and, as well as being closely and irrefutably linked to premature death, being seriously overweight is an almost certain guarantee that you'll suffer from a range of other health problems.

These include degenerative arthritis in any, and sometimes all, of the weight bearing joints – ankles, knees, hips and lumbar spine – back pain, disc problems, haemorrhoids, high blood pressure, high cholesterol, increased risk of heart disease and stroke, varicose veins, foot problems and breathing difficulties.

Being seriously overweight has social consequences, too, the main one being that it restricts sporting activities, which also leads to a gradual decline in overall fitness and yet more weight gain. For many people, being seriously overweight also carries a heavy emotional burden and can lead to psychological disturbance. Relationship problems, lack of self-esteem, poor self-image – all these can combine to reduce the enjoyment of life both in social and employment terms.

Apart from plain bad eating, one of the key factors in obesity is basic metabolic rate (BMR). This is the efficiency with which your resting body can burn up the fuel which you consume as food – and it's the reason why, say, two brothers living in the same home and eating exactly the same food can have totally different body shapes, one fat, one thin. The percentage of brown fat in the body is also thought to be significant. This brown fat is able to store huge amounts of energy without causing obesity and people whose bodies have a smaller percentage of brown fat turn their surplus energy into white fat.

While there are some glandular disorders which cause weight gain, they're comparatively rare and usually treatable. Thyroid disorders are probably the most common. Steroid drugs, oral contraceptives, HRT (hormone replacement therapy) and insulin used by diabetics may cause weight gain, too. But the vast majority of overweight people pile it on simply because they consume more calories than they burn.

Of all the multitude of weight reducing treatments, the only one that really works is permanently to change the way you eat. Slimming pills, injections, liposuction, crash diets and 'miracle cures' are usually expensive, frequently hazardous to your health and never work long term.

Low calorie diets don't work either because your metabolism slows down to conserve energy as you reduce your calorie input. At the end of a week or so of 800, 900 or 1,000 calorie-a-day consumption you feel tired, irritable and desperate. A two-day binge puts back all the weight you lost and you're set on a life of yo-yo dieting.

American Professor of Nutrition, Judith Stern, maintains that the overweight pear shape is at less risk of heart disease than the overweight barrel shape. Every time the pear loses weight quickly and puts it on again, it shifts up the body a little, and eventually the pear becomes a barrel, has lost no weight overall and is at greater risk of heart disease.

Check your own waist/hip ratio. Measure your waist around the belly button, then round the biggest part of your hips. Then divide the waist measurement by the hip measurement. For women the result should be 0.75 or less and for men 1.0 or less. As the figure goes up, your risk of heart disease increases, too.

Garbology is a new science which can show us how little people understand about government-inspired healthy eating messages. American archaeologists have recently started to study garbage tips and by using core extractors they take samples from infill sites all around the US, which they can date very accurately from layers of newspaper.

When the US Government recommended a reduction of animal fat to avoid bowel cancer, the garbage tips overflowed with all the fat that had been cut off bacon, steaks and joints. But within weeks the garbologists were finding a dramatic increase in wrappers from processed meat products like salamis, sausages and bologna.

The next Government advice to protect against cancer was 'eat more green vegetables' and supermarket sales boomed. Unfortunately, much more was sold than eaten and the garbologists found tons of uncooked, uneaten green vegetables in the garbage tips. There's no point in buying it unless you eat it.

All the ideal height and weight charts are based on averages and many of them from quite long out-of-date insurance company actuarial tables. I believe the margin of error is greater than generally accepted because weight isn't the only measure of health and fitness. Spiritual and emotional health are difficult to measure, but play an enormous part in your total wellbeing. Peace of mind and a positive attitude increase the body's natural resistance and resilience and I'm certain that being 10 per cent overweight and happy is far better than striving to get 10 per cent underweight and being miserable. In fact, life expectancy statistics confirm this.

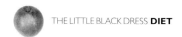

As an approximate guide here's a chart of relative height and weight measurements – 10–15 per cent above the indicated weight and you may consider doing something about it, 20–30 per cent above and you should take some action.

WOMEN	HEIGHT	MEN
Weight without clothes	Without shoes	Weight without clothes
	1.95m/6ft4in	181lb/80.4kg
	1.92m/6ft3in	176lb/78.2kg
	1.89m/6ft2in	171lb/76kg
	1.87m/6ft1in	166lb/73.8kg
152lb/67.6kg	1.84m/6ft	162lb/72kg
148lb/65.8kg	1.81m/5ft11in	158lb/70.2kg
144lb/64kg	1.78m/5ft10in	153lb/68kg
140lb/62.2kg	1.76m/5ft9in	149lb/66.2kg
136lb/60.4kg	1.73m/5ft8in	145lb/64.4kg
132lb/58.7kg	1.70m/5ft7in	140lb/62.2kg
128lb/56.9kg	1.68m/5ft6in	136lb/60.4kg
123lb/54.7kg	1.65m/5ft5in	133lb/59.1kg
120lb/53.3kg	1.62m/5ft4in	130lb/57.7kg
116lb/52.4kg	1.60m/5ft3in	127lb/56.4kg
113lb/50.2kg	1.57m/5ft2in	123lb/54.7kg
110lb/49kg	1.55m/5ft1in	
107lb/47.6kg	1.52m/5ft	

BODY MASS INDEX - BMI

Body Mass Index is a universally standard way of calculating the relationship between height and weight. To work out your own BMI, divide your weight in kilograms by your height in metres squared. This calculation is known at Quetelet's Index:–

$$BMI = \frac{\text{Weight in kilograms}}{\text{Height in metres}^2}$$

The resulting number is an excellent guide – anything between 20 and 25 is within the ideal weight range, 25–30 is overweight, 30–40 is moderately obese and over 40 is grossly obese. These figures are based on the American Metropolitan Life Insurance calculations.

In the UK, Government figures show a continuing increase in the amount of obesity (BMI greater than 30) and overweight (BMI over 25) since the 1980s. The average weight of men has increased by around 1kg/2lb between the ages of 16–49, and 3kg/6lb between the ages of 50–64. By 1993 the number of men in Britain who were overweight had gone up by 44 per cent and the women by 30 per cent. The number of seriously obese Britons doubled between 1980 and 1993, rising from 6 to 13 per cent of men, and from 8 to 16 per cent of women.

In 2001 the appalling truth is that 50 per cent of the entire population is sufficiently overweight to be a potential medical hazard and one person in five in the UK is clinically obese. Changing eating patterns, the overwhelming dominance of the food market by convenience food manufacturers, food processors and the take-away giants, together with the nut, crisp, snack and confectionery manufacturers and their multi-billion pound advertising budgets have turned us into a nation of junk food eaters.

Combine this with the ever-increasing decline of physical activity in all age groups, from the youngest children at school to retired pensioners, and there is an ever-widening gap between the calories we consume and the calories we burn. Add to this the poor nutritional value that's wrapped around the junk food calories, the fact that an average of 45 per cent of all our calories come from fats, with a consequent decline in our use of all the complex carbohydrates in traditional starchy foods like wholemeal bread, brown rice, potatoes, oats and other cereals and pasta, and we have the recipe for a 21st-century health and nutrition catastrophe.

So much of the advice about nutrition is conflicting and confusing. That's because a lot of it is promoted by commercial companies who have a vested interest in making their types of food, range of products, pills or services sound healthier than everyone else's. With the exception of following a good vegetarian regime or an extremely careful vegan diet, any nutritional advice which removes entire food groups from your diet should be treated with great suspicion.

Avoiding all dairy products, all wheat or other cereal foods, cutting out all carbohydrates and eating masses of animal protein isn't the route to good health or sensible weight loss. Though real food allergies can be serious and life threatening, they're comparatively rare and cannot be accurately diagnosed by a machine in a chemist's or a health food store, by dangling a pendulum on a piece of string or by the 'vibrations' of your voice over the telephone. Adverse food reactions or intolerance are more common, but the same reservations about questionable tests still apply. (You can check for yourself – see Exclusion Diets on page 40.)

It might seem complicated, but by following the 'wheel of health' guidelines on page 21, you can build a week's eating that suits your taste and lifestyle.

FAT, LOW-FAT AND NO FAT

The world has gone mad. Everyone is obsessed by fat in their diets, which of course makes them easy targets for the unscrupulous food industry. Almost every package has screaming labels saying things like 98 per cent fat free – and they're often on food which don't contain fats anyway, like breakfast cereals and bread. I'm amazed that no-one has yet marketed a '100 per cent fat free' mineral water – but I'm sure it's only a matter of time. I see women in my clinic who are so obsessed with fat that they can tell you the fat content of every product on the supermarket shelves by heart, and their idea of low-fat means no fat at all.

It's certainly true that most of us get far too many calories from fat – the average being around 45 per cent, when it should be less than 35 per cent. Here's what you need to know to maintain a healthy balance. Cut down on as much of the saturated animal fat as you can. You don't need it and it's one of the main causes of blocked arteries and heart disease. Remove all visible fat from meat and poultry. Don't eat the skin on roast chicken, duck or goose. No matter how tempting, throw away the crackling from roast pork. Manufactured meat products contain horrendous amounts of saturated fat and 85 per cent of the calories they provide come from this lethal ingredient. They include sausages, salami, pâté, meat pies and pasties, scotch eggs and doner kebabs – although the traditional shish kebab on a skewer is fine.

Dairy products are another rich source of saturated fats, but you can choose lower fat versions of cheeses. Most people don't realise that, with the exception of cream cheese, soft cheeses have less fat than hard cheeses. In fact, the harder the cheese the higher the fat content. You really can enjoy that really runny Brie, and for women, a matchbox-sized piece of cheese a day is an essential source of bone-building calcium. There's also no need to be fanatical about milk and

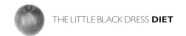

yoghurt. Even full-cream Jersey milk is 96 per cent fat free and switching to watery, tasteless skimmed milk saves very little fat and deprives you of much needed vitamin D. Never give skimmed or semi-skimmed milk to children under five – they need those precious calories.

Cakes and biscuits are an unexpected source of saturated fat. It's not just the high sugar content that's bad for slimmers. Few people realise that palm oil and coconut oil also contain high levels of saturated fat – which is why it's so important to read the labels on any food products you buy. Both these oils are cheap and widely used in the food processing industry, but you might as well put dripping on your bread for all the good they do you. Also, by the way, dripping made at home tastes a hell of a lot better.

Margarines are all factory-made industrial products which contain a host of chemicals as well as trans-fats, which are as bad for your heart as saturated fats.

Mono-unsaturated fats like olive oil and other nut and seed oils have a double benefit They don't cause any harm and they help the body to eliminate cholesterol. Like all fats, they contain around 900 calories per 100g/4oz, so just because they're healthy, don't eat too much of them. But on no account avoid them completely.

Poly-unsaturated fats can be good or bad, depending on the balance between omega-3 and omega-6 fatty acids They're all better than saturated or trans-fats – and although sunflower seed oil and corn oil are reasonable choice, rapeseed, safflower and flaxseed are the best.

The conventional advice from both the British and American health departments is to follow the healthy eating pyramid which virtually eliminates all fats except small amounts of poly-unsaturates. This flies in the face of all the evidence discovered by studying the 'Mediterranean' diet, which has proved to be so much more healthy than the eating patterns anywhere else in the Western world.

The most recent scientific studies have shown that even though both of these types of diet help reduce levels of the dangerous LDL form of cholesterol, only the Mediterranean diet, rich in olive oil, garlic, fish, fruit and vegetables, actually improved the condition of already damaged arteries.

Low-fat doesn't mean no fat – and you must remember that there is a whole group of fats known as essential fatty acids. No matter how much you need to lose weight, you must always include oily fish, olive oil, flaxseed oil and modest amounts of the other nut and seed oils in your diet unless your weight loss is going to be at the expense of your long-term health.

HOW TO BALANCE YOUR DIET SO IT LOOKS GOOD, TASTES GOOD AND DOES YOU GOOD

The wheel of health is divided into three equal segments, one of which is then split into two smaller equal segments and a third much smaller still. Plan your shopping and eating around these proportions and you'll be amazed at how simple it is.

Segment A

Include all the wonderful fruits, vegetables and salads, get at least five portions a day and a good mixture. It may sound a lot but it's only about 500g/1lb in weight. Fruit or vegetable juice counts as a portion. An apple, pear or orange, a small bunch of grapes, an average portion of any cooked or raw vegetable, a small bowl of salad, all count as one portion. So, a glass of orange juice with breakfast, an apple midmorning, a pitta bread stuffed with humus and mixed salad at lunchtime, broccoli and carrots with your evening meal and a bunch of grapes and a pear during the evening, gets you up to seven!

Segment B

These starchy foods should provide half your daily calories. Have plenty of wholemeal bread, rolls, chapatis, breakfast cereals, particularly muesli, porridge, Shredded Wheat, Weetabix and others low in added salt and sugar. Include, too, pasta, rice, noodles, potatoes – steamed, boiled or baked and sweet potatoes – and lots of beans, chickpeas and lentils – canned are fine, but rinse well to remove salt. Contrary to old-fashioned dieting ideas, and even the latest gimmick slimming books, these starchy foods aren't fattening.

Segment C1

This should consist of protein - lean beef, pork, lamb or poultry, all types of fish, offal, eggs, more beans, lentils, chickpeas, nuts (not salted or chocolate covered), seeds and vegetarian meat substitutes like textured vegetable protein, Quorn, tofu and other soy products These, like the dairy foods in segment C2, should be taken in modest quantities and should be eaten steamed, baked, grilled or roasted on a rack to reduce fat content.

Segment C2

This should be dairy products - milk, cheese, yoghurt, fromage frais. They're all available in low and very low fat versions, but it's worth remembering that even full fat milk is just under 4 per cent fat - a pork sausage is 32 per cent fat. Skimmed and semi-skimmed milk should not be given to children under five. Although these dairy products form a small portion of your total food, they're important sources of calcium.

Segment C3

This is by far the smallest group and should represent the lowest contribution to your total daily calories. These are the high-fat, high-sugar foods which are often the treats we all enjoy. Don't cut them out, you'll be miserable, just be a bit mean. Butter, margarine, low fat spreads, cooking oils, mayonnaise, and other oily salad dressings should all be used sparingly. But my advice is always to avoid margarine of any sort. After all, how can something made in a factory compare with the natural flavours of real butter, preferably organic and unsalted? Watch out, too, for anything labelled vegetable oil as this is almost certain to contain either coconut or palms oil, which are both high in saturated fats, the sort which clog your arteries and raise your cholesterol.

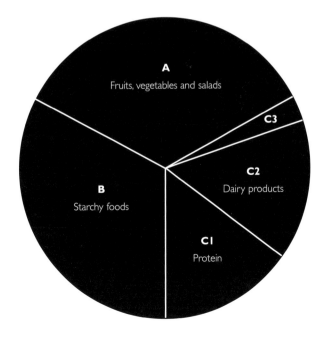

A
Fruits, vegetables and salads

C3

C2
Dairy products

B
Starchy foods

C1
Protein

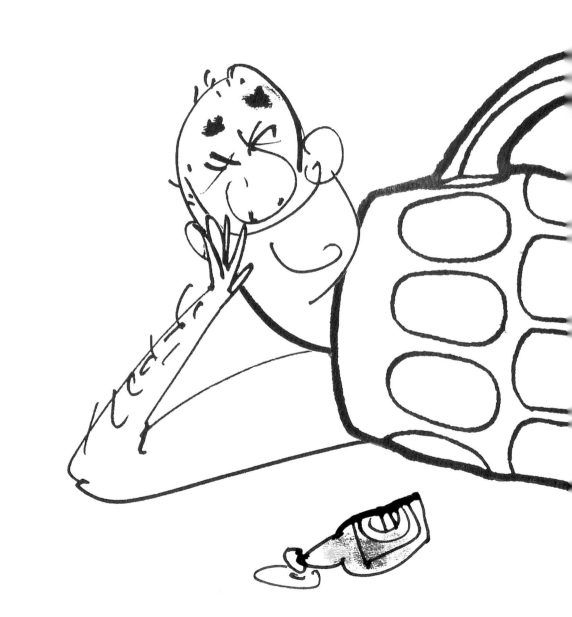

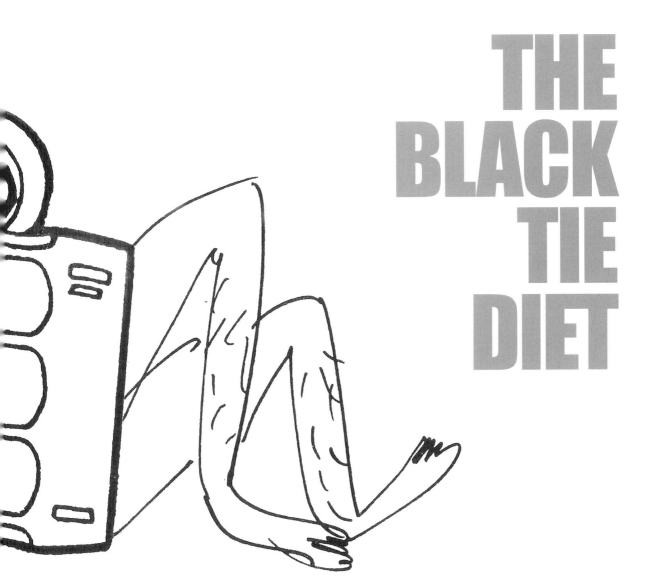

THE BLACK TIE DIET

Unless your job demands it, it's unlikely that most of you have to wear a black tie with your DJ very often. But when an invitation drops on your doormat and you see the dreaded words 'Black Tie' under the dress requirements, does your heart sink? Will your belly button be poking its way through the gaping spaces of your dress shirt? Has your wife wickedly and perversely shrunk it's collar size from the original 16? Will you have to dash out and buy a cummerbund to hide the fact that you can't do up the waist buttons on the trousers and the zip keeps sliding down?

Disaster!

Don't despair. As much as the Little Black Dress Diet will help women with their predicament, the Black Tie Diet will solve yours and you won't end up rushing out at the last minute to buy a new DJ or hire one. Nor will you have to decline the invitation.

This diet is a ten-day blitz especially designed for men and though it works this is not a healthy option for your long term eating habits. The plan is definitely for carnivores as it's based on a high protein low carbohydrate intake because the majority of men prefer eating meat and any weight loss regime which forces them into vegetarianism or at best a

life of endless salads is doomed to failure. If you are a veggie simply substitute the meat recipes for high protein veggie alternatives like beans, lentils, chickpeas, tofu or manufactured soy products. The diet will not work if you eat vast amounts of cheese as your main protein food, as this will push your fat intake to astronomical levels.

You must make sure that you consume at least 2 litres/3-3$\frac{1}{2}$ pints of fluid each day, half of which should be still mineral water with an added measure of Pure Plan. Take two teaspoons of the Swiss herbal elixir BioStrath in the morning and another two in the evening. This combination boosts your metabolism, assuages your appetite and stimulates all of the body's eliminative functions.

Throw away the salt cellar – it's bad for your blood pressure and encourages fluid retention. Instead use all the wonderful herbs and spices to flavour your food. As a bonus, many of these will actually help with your weight loss plan. If you don't cheat you will easily lose 4-5kg/10lb in 10 days and it's quite safe to repeat this diet four times a year. If you need to lose substantially more than 3kg/7lb then long term you must choose one of the other healthier eating options in this book.

DAY 1

Breakfast: 2 poached eggs with 2 poached tomatoes and 2 rashers of lean grilled unsmoked bacon.
1 large glass of grapefruit juice.
1 cup of tea or coffee without sugar.

Main Meal: Italian Steak in Red Wine (page 67).
Peas, broccoli and mushrooms.
Large bunch of grapes.
1 glass of wine.

Light Meal: Watercress Salad (page 90).
2 brown rice cakes.
Pear.

DAY 2

Breakfast: 2 low fat grilled sausages, grilled tomatoes, grilled mushrooms.
Glass of tomato juice.
1 cup of tea or coffee.

Main Meal: half a small melon.
Chicken and Vegetable Stir-Fry (page 67).
Soaked dried fruits and low-fat live yoghurt mixed with lemon zest, a teaspoon of honey and fresh mint.
1 glass of wine.

Light Meal: large bowl of Fruity, Spicy Carrot Soup (page 100).
2 rice cakes.
Bunch of grapes.

DAY 3

Breakfast: half a fresh pink grapefruit.
Large helping of baked beans on 1 thick slice of unbuttered wholemeal toast.
Glass of unsalted mixed vegetable juice.
1 cup of tea or coffee.

Main Meal: half an avocado with My One and Only Dressing (page 93).
Herby Herrings (page 70).
A large red onion and tomato salad, drizzled with olive oil, lemon juice and lots of black pepper.
Small portion of Brie or similar soft cheese.
1 apple, 1 pear.
1 glass of wine.

Light Meal: Beetroot Booster Salad (page 89).
1 ripe banana.

DAY 4

Breakfast: poached smoked haddock with poached tomatoes.
1 cup of tea or coffee.
glass of orange juice.

Main Meal: small green salad with Five-Flavour Olive Oil and Vinegar Dressing (page 94).
Indian Mushrooms and Prawns (page 72).
Large portion of fresh fruit salad.
1 glass of wine.

Light Meal: scrambled eggs and smoked salmon (or Superbrunch – page 60).
2 rice cakes and a small carton of plain live yoghurt.

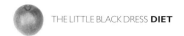
DAY 5

Breakfast: large bowl porridge made with skimmed milk.
Glass of orange juice.
I cup of tea or coffee.

Main Meal: fresh melon.
Grilled Spiced Chicken (page 76).
Mixed raw vegetable salad (carrot, courgette, peppers, celery, broccoli,
cauliflower, cucumber, tomato) with a drizzle of olive oil.
Large slice of fresh pineapple.
I glass of wine.

Light Meal: 2 thick slices unbuttered, wholemeal toast covered in thin
slices of low-fat cheddar cheese, sprinkled with Worcestershire sauce
and put under a hot grill till the cheese melts.
I large tomato.
Breakfast Compôte (page 63), sprinkled with sunflower and pumpkin
seeds.

DAY 6

Breakfast: fresh melon.
3 thin slices ham with all fat removed, I poached egg, I tomato,
Glass of orange juice.
I cup of tea or coffee.

Main Meal: Spanish Rabbit (page 75), served with plain boiled
potatoes liberally sprinkled with chopped parsley.
A mix of chopped dried dates and apricots with natural live yoghurt.
I glass of wine.

Light Meal: Three-Colour Coleslaw (page 87).
A small portion of Brie or similar soft cheese.

2 rice cakes.
I glass of apple juice.

DAY 7

Breakfast: Fish for Brains (page 110) with
2 large tomatoes.
Glass of unsalted vegetable juice.
I cup of tea or coffee.

Main Meal: Garlicious Soup (page 98).
Aromatic Lamb (page 73), with 2 green vegetables.
Mixed berries – strawberries, blackberries, blueberries, raspberries.
I glass of wine.

Light Meal: Bread and Tomato Salad (page 86).
I glass of apple juice.
A banana and I tablespoon of mixed sunflower and pumpkin seeds
and pine nuts.

DAY 8

Breakfast: half a pink grapefruit.
2 boiled eggs.
I thin slice unbuttered wholemeal toast.
I cup of tea or coffee.

Main Meal: Prawn and Mushroom Bake (page 72)
with Watercress salad (page90).
a large ripe peach.
I glass of wine.

Light Meal:
Chinese Stir-Fry Surprise Soup (page 99).
low-fat natural yoghurt with a little honey and a pinch of cinnamon

DAY 9

Breakfast: a pair of undyed kippers – to avoid the smell of cooking these delicious and nutritious fish, put them head first into a large jug, fill with boiling water, tightly cover with foil and leave for 10 minutes. Remove foil and enjoy.

1 glass of orange juice.

1 cup of tea or coffee.

Main Meal: Beery Stew (page 74).

small piece of Brie or other soft cheese with a stick of celery – eat the leaves.

1 glass of wine.

Light Meal: Warm Salad of Mushrooms and Radicchio (page 88).

2 rice cakes.

1 glass of pineapple juice.

DAY 10

Breakfast: 2 fried eggs, 2 rashers lean grilled unsmoked bacon, 2 grilled tomatoes – but these are fried eggs with a difference. Put a large plate on top of a pan of boiling water, when the plate's too hot to touch break the eggs on to it while the bacon and tomatoes are cooking. They'll all be ready together and you've got fried eggs with no added fat.

1 glass of mixed orange and grapefruit juice.

1 cup of tea or coffee.

Main Meal: salad of sliced onions and tomatoes with a drizzle of olive oil.

Steamed Salmon with Lemon and Fennel (page 79),

with plain boiled brown rice.

any fruit sorbet sprinkled with chopped mixed nuts or chopped dried

fruits – both if you like but not too much.

1 glass of wine.

Light Meal:

Large bowl of Curried Pumpkin Soup (page 101).

a selection of any fresh fruits.

You're going to look terrific in your black tie and DJ and whoever's wearing the little black dress will be proud of you. It's okay to switch the days around or have the meals in any order that suits your lifestyle. What you can't do is to mix meals from different days. I've said it before, and I'm going to say it again, no matter how much weight you lose you should not repeat this diet for at least two or three months. High protein diets are not a long term healthy option, but fine for an occasional short burst.

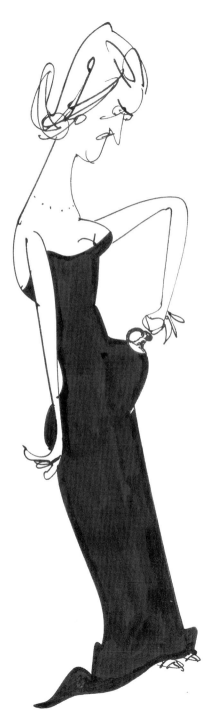

24 HOURS TO BEAT THE BLOAT

Slinky, clingy frocks are all the rage – and don't they look great? That is, of course, until you look in the mirror the night before the posh frock outing and a bulge resembling the later stages of pregnancy has suddenly appeared where your flat tummy was the day before.

What do you do? Panic, ring up your host and plead illness, dig out your old maternity dress or wear a kaftan, look up liposuction in the Yellow Pages – there's no need. You can beat the bloat with this easy and effective 24-hour plan.

The most common of causes is fluid retention and that may be because a period is due, or you've had an over-indulgence of salt from burger bar, French fries, or maybe you've pigged out on all those salty nibbles at the office party.

Wind or constipation can also be uncomfortable reasons for your dilemma. An excessive amount of wind may be trapped in your stomach or lower down in your small or large intestine, your large bowel may be full as a result of constipation and frequently these two factors go together.

If 'bloated belly syndrome' (BBS) is something that you know happens to you from time to time, be prepared and make sure you have the necessary ingredients at home to solve your problem in time for the big night out.

BEAT THE BLOAT - THE ACTION PLAN

The night before your outing take a good look in the mirror and at the first sign of BBS drink 2 large glasses of hot water with a slice of lemon. This will stimulate your kidneys and start the process of fluid elimination. Take half a cube of Ortisan, a natural fruit jelly which is a very gentle and effective laxative, to relieve any constipation.

Put a tablespoon of chopped parsley and a teaspoon of crushed dill seeds into a glass, add boiling water, stir well, cover and leave to stand for 10 minutes. Pour through a strainer and sip slowly just before bed. The parsley is a gentle diuretic and the dill seeds help the elimination of existing wind and prevent more from forming. You may be up two or three times in the night to go to the loo, but it's worth it to get rid of BBS, and you can always cover the shadows under your eyes with make-up.

First thing in the morning take another large glass of hot water with lemon, and the other half of the Ortisan cube. For breakfast have a small bowl of porridge made with half a cup of oats, half a cup of skimmed milk, a cup of water and no salt. With your breakfast take a small pot of Yakult and a sachet of Beneflora, both of which supply essential good bacteria which make your digestion more efficient.

At lunch time eat an apple, a generous bunch of grapes and a ripe banana – make sure the skin is just going speckly brown. Have another glass of hot water with lemon.

During the afternoon drink at least 2 cups of fennel tea which you can get in teabags from health stores and most supermarkets, or use the baby drink granules, and eat 6 dates – the semi-dried ones in plastic containers, not the sugary ones in wooden boxes. Fennel is a powerful anti-gas herb and the dates provide good fibre and lots of iron to set you up for the evening.

When you get home have another glass of parsley tea and a small teacup of slippery elm food which you can buy in any health store – mix a teaspoonful into a paste with a little cold water, top up with boiling water and a teaspoon of honey and drink slowly. It's an effective antacid and digestive protector which will leave your stomach feeling soothed, relaxed and comfortable.

If you have a real disaster and your stomach suddenly swells up in the afternoon of your posh frock date, swing into the emergency action plan. Take 2 tablets of the natural diuretic Aqualette (from health stores and pharmacies), which is made from dandelion and horsetail, for rapid loss of retained fluid, and a couple of charcoal tablets which will absorb any trapped wind.

Have a long soak in a hot bath to which you've added 5 drops of peppermint oil mixed with a dessetspoonful of grape seed or sunflower seed oil. Peppermint is not only invigorating but also a wonderful digestive aid, and you will absorb some through your skin.

Your slinky outfit will fit you like a glove without a sign of BBS. But take care if you're going out for dinner. Avoid the pre-meal nibbles, choose sensible dishes which are not too bulky, fish is easier to digest than fillet steak or roast beef. Say no to the rolls and butter, and don't ruin the effect by finishing with sticky toffee pudding which will sit like a stone on your stomach.

Remember that mint is a perfect way to end your meal but not covered in chocolate – virtually any restaurant will be able to provide you with some mint tea after your dinner but don't be tempted to add milk – it's disgusting.

Natalie Wood

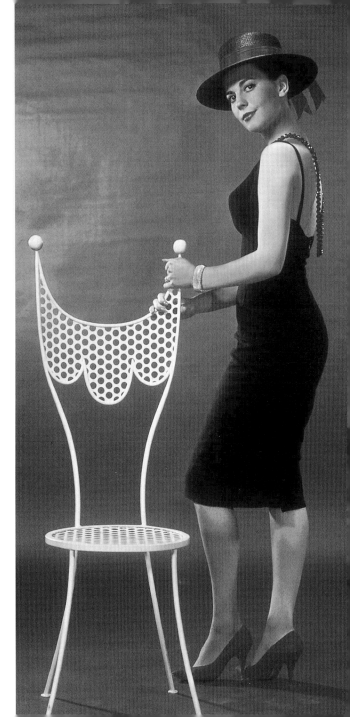

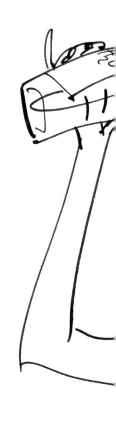

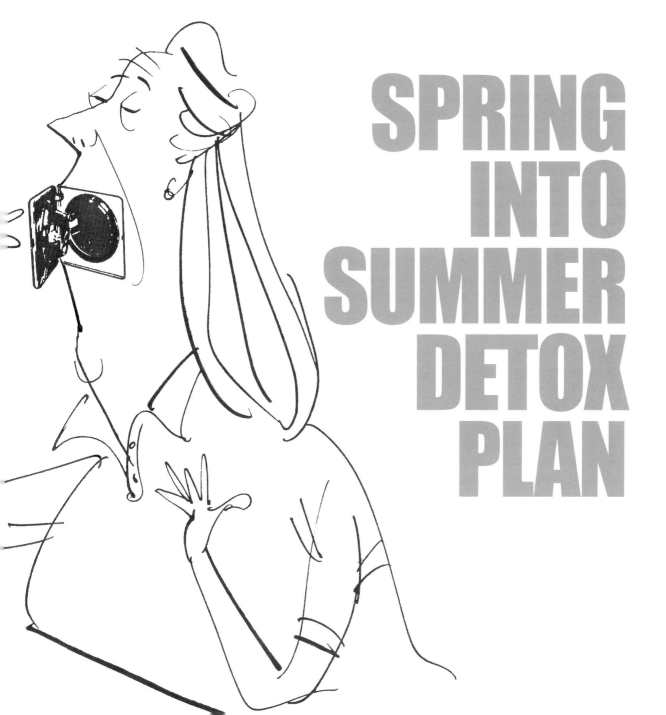

SPRING INTO SUMMER DETOX PLAN

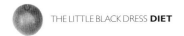

Are you panicking? Do the thoughts of summer holidays, beaches and bikinis fill you with horror? Now's the time to boost vitality, raise defences and shed that excess baggage, in just seven short days. This one-week eating plan is a three-pronged attack:-

1 A short, sharp fast kicks off the detoxifying process. Because there's little bulk in the first 48 hours, unfriendly bacteria starve to death in your intestine, releasing toxins which may cause headaches. Drink plenty of fluids and they'll go away.

2 An abundance of immune-boosting foods, increasing natural resistance to invading bacteria and viruses, to protect you from winter infections.

3   The low-fat and high-starch content rests the liver and encourages the brain's production of 'feel-good' chemicals that fight winter fatigue and depression.

This meat-free week gives you massive quantities of protective vitamins and minerals. A, C and E, betacarotene and the other powerful anti-cancer carotenoids, zinc and selenium that protect against heart disease and infections, as well as cancer, and the enormous health benefits of garlic.

ELIMINATING AND RESISTANCE-BOOSTING SUPPLEMENTS

This is not a diet for life, but a short sharp shock which you can use three or four times a year. To speed elimination, each morning add 15ml of Pure Plan (from health stores) – a wonderful mixture of dandelion, burdock, artichoke, fennel, seaweed, wild pansy and tamarind – to 1 litre/1 1/3 pints of still mineral water. Drink the whole bottle during the day.

To compensate for any vitamin shortfall take a daily Genesis multivitamin pill (health stores). Take 2 teaspoons of the Swiss herbal tonic Bio-Strath Elixir (health stores and chemists) 3 times daily – it boosts white cells and natural resistance.

DAY 1

A real fasting day. Drink loads of water and herbal teas throughout the day.

Breakfast, lunch and evening meal are the same: 1 glass of unsweetened fruit or salt free vegetable juice plus a carton of natural live yoghurt. Try to start this diet on a non-working quiet day – don't worry, it can only get better!

DAY 2

Breakfast: This is the **standard breakfast** you'll eat for the rest of the week. I portion fresh fruit – vary throughout the week, apple, pear, mango, grapes, pineapple, grapefruit – plus 2 slices of wholemeal toast spread with low-fat cottage cheese, a carton of low-fat live yoghurt, a small glass of skimmed milk and a cup of herb or weak Indian tea without milk or sugar.

Lunch: I kiwi fruit, 200g/7oz mixed raw vegetable salad – a bed of iceberg lettuce, filled with grated carrot, celeriac and beetroot, with a squeeze of lemon juice and a drizzle of olive oil – plus 175g/6oz of any steamed vegetables, sprinkled with a chopped clove of garlic and a drizzle of olive oil. Herb or weak Indian tea.

Supper: 50g/2oz blueberries in 100g/4oz unsweetened muesli mixed with a tablespoon of orange juice and a carton of low fat live yoghurt, herb or weak Indian tea.

DAY 3

Standard breakfast

Lunch: large mango, 175g/6oz mixed salad, including watercress, fresh mint, spring onions, tomato, red and yellow peppers, chicory, baby spinach and beansprouts. A lemon juice and olive oil dressing. Plus I large jacket potato with 50g/2oz low fat fromage frais whipped with chopped chives and a clove of garlic. Vegetable juice.

Supper: carton of low-fat live yoghurt mixed with blackberries, blueberries and I teaspoonful of honey. I crusty wholemeal roll with a matchbox-sized piece of soft cheese – Brie, Camembert or similar. Herb or weak Indian tea.

DAY 4

This is a very special day where your main food will be rice. Like fasting, rice days are traditionally used by naturopaths as a cleansing treatment. Start by preparing the rice for the whole day. You'll need 270g/9oz dry brown rice cooked in 1.7 litres/3 pints of water. If you prefer, cook half the rice in half the water and the other half in vegetable stock for a more savoury flavour.

Breakfast: 90g/3oz cooked rice with 150g/5oz stewed apple flavoured with honey, cinnamon and grated lemon rind.

Lunch: 90g/3oz cooked rice with 200g/7oz steamed vegetables – celery, leek, carrot, tomato, spinach, broccoli and shredded cabbage.

Supper: 90g/3oz rice mixed with soaked dried apricots, raisins, sultanas, and the flesh of a pink grapefruit.
Drink only water today.

DAY 5

Standard breakfast.

Lunch: I apple, I pear, 175g/6oz raw vegetable salad – cauliflower and broccoli florets, carrot, spring onion, grated red cabbage, mange tout – tossed in olive oil and cider vinegar dressing, sprinkled with a teaspoon of raisins and 3 chopped brazil nuts. Large jacket potato filled with 90g/3oz steamed spinach chopped with 2 teaspoons of olive oil, clove of garlic and a generous grating of nutmeg. Herb or weak Indian tea.

Supper: 90g/3oz fromage frais mixed with a carton of low-fat live yoghurt, poured over a generous bowl of mixed fruit salad, including kiwi, pineapple, orange, grapes, blueberries, apple. Cup of herb tea.

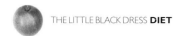

DAY 6

Standard breakfast

Lunch: Banana, 175g/6oz mixed salad – shredded iceberg lettuce and one dark green or red lettuce, tomato, olives, red pepper, carrot, spring onions, cucumber, a clove of garlic, fennel and watercress – with a dressing of lemon juice, walnut oil and tarragon. Plus a large jacket potato with 90g/3oz steamed French or runner beans with a dessertspoon of sunflower oil sprinkled with finely chopped onions. Herb or weak Indian tea.

Supper: 90g/3oz muesli mixed with a dessertspoon lemon juice, teaspoon honey, grated apple, carton of low-fat live yoghurt. 1 slice wholemeal bread with a matchbox-sized piece of Brie, Camembert or similar soft cheese. 1 slice wholemeal bread with honey. Cup of tea.

DAY 7

Standard breakfast

Lunch: 175g/6oz mixed salad – watercress, baby spinach, mixed lettuce leaves, parsley, celery, garlic, chives, basil, tomato – with a dressing of equal parts of walnut oil, olive oil and cider vinegar and a teaspoon of Dijon mustard, sprinkled with sunflower seeds. 90g/3oz boiled potatoes and EITHER trout stuffed with finely chopped parsley, onion, tomato and pine nuts, covered in thinly sliced lemon, baked in foil with a little olive oil, OR vegetarian alternative – stir-fried tofu with shredded carrot, beansprouts, mange tout and soy sauce OR a grilled vegeburger. A glass of dry white wine.

Supper: A whole pink grapefruit, 2 poached free-range eggs on 2 slices of wholemeal toast with a scrape of butter. A cup of herb or weak Indian tea.

Well done. If you haven't cheated you're probably 1.8-2kg/4-5lb lighter, your eyes are bright, skin clear and you feel terrific. The high fibre content of this week has really got your digestion working and all the super-protective natural chemicals in pure, unadulterated food have lifted your spirits physically and mentally.

Taking some exercise is really vital and no matter what the weather, dress appropriately and get yourself into the fresh air and daylight whenever possible. Even on an overcast day enough light will get into your eyes to help ward off the awful problems of SAD (seasonal affective disorder). A brisk 20-minute walk three times a week will make all the difference. For a terrific extra vitality boost, drink these vitality juices regularly – a juice machine is probably the best health investment you can make.

BLUE BY YOU

100g/4oz blueberries, 3 passionfruit, 1 medium Cantaloupe melon, 1 mango.
A juice guaranteed to chase away the blues and put a glow on your skin, this tonic-in-a-glass will give you instant energy and super immunity. A magical mixture that's better than turning water into wine.

PARSLEY, SAGE, ROSEMARY AND . . .

4 carrots, 3 sticks celery, handful parsley, 6 sage leaves, 2 teaspoons rosemary leaves removed from stalk, small sprig thyme.
Just like Simon and Garfunkel's memorable song, this juice is the ideal combination of vital force and calming influences. It's a gentle giant as it nourishes body, mind and spirit.

ROOT JUICE

I small beetroot with leaves, 3 carrots, 2 apples

Vitality depends on every cell in the body being fed by your blood. If it's not in peak condition it won't perform this function efficiently and vitality flags. This vitality juice builds healthier blood and provides essential ingredients for cell protection.

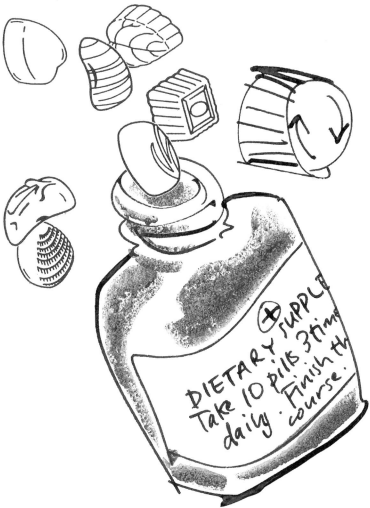

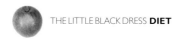

THREE-DAY DETOX DIET

This three-day plan is pretty low in calories and you will feel hungry from time to time. Don't spoil the effect by cheating. You won't be drinking coffee, and only very weak tea without milk or sugar, so your caffeine intake comes to an abrupt halt. The combination of less food, no coffee and the effects of detoxification will almost certainly cause a headache. Drink masses of water and try to avoid pain killers. The headache is transient and you are going to feel absolutely great by day four and you'll be full of the protective antioxidants you need.

Do the first two days when your workload is at its lightest. To help overcome the hunger pangs take two teaspoons of the Swiss herbal tonic BioStrath elixir three times a day and, if you don't have a juicer, Biotta Organic vegetable juices are salt-free, delicious and available from good health stores.

DAY 1

Kick start your metabolism with Day 1 of the Detox Plan. More than your daily needs of potassium, vitamins B1, B6, folic acid, niacin, A, C and E – the powerful and protective antioxidants.

Breakfast: an orange, half a grapefruit, a large slice of melon.
A glass of unsalted vegetable juice.
A cup of herb tea with honey.

Midday: a plateful of raw red and yellow peppers, cucumber, tomato, broccoli, cauliflower, celery, carrots, radishes and lots of fresh parsley.
Add extra virgin olive oil and lemon juice.
A large glass of unsweetened fruit juice.

Evening meal: large mixed salad with extra virgin olive oil and lemon juice. Lettuce, tomato, watercress, onion, garlic, beetroot, celeriac, fresh mint and any herbs you like.
A large glass of unsweetened fruit juice or unsalted vegetable juice.
Drink at least four pints of fluid – water, weak black tea or herb tea – each day.

DAY 2

More than you need of phosphorus, magnesium, potassium, copper, vitamin B1, B6, folic acid, vitamins A, C and E, and a good supply of protein, calcium, fibre, iron and selenium.

Breakfast: a large glass of hot water, a thick slice of lemon, a dessertspoon of honey. A carton of natural low-fat live yogurt.

Mid morning: a large glass of vegetable juice, a handful each of raisins, dried apricots and fresh nuts.

Lunch: a salad of grated carrot, red cabbage, apple with sliced red pepper, tomato, radishes, celery, a sprinkle of sunflower seeds, lemon juice and olive oil.
A cup of herb or weak Indian tea with honey, no milk.

Mid-afternoon: a glass of fruit juice and a banana.

Evening meal: any 3 cooked vegetables (not potatoes) with olive oil, nutmeg and lemon juice.
A cup of herb tea or weak Indian tea.

During the evening: a mixture of dried fruits and unsalted nuts and as much fresh fruit as you like.

DAY 3

More than your day's requirements of fibre, phosphorus, magnesium, potassium, copper; B1, B2, niacin, B6, folic acid, vitamins A, C and E. Lots of vitamin B12, calcium and iron.

Breakfast: fresh fruit salad of apple, pear, grapes, mango and pineapple, with a carton of live yoghurt and a tablespoon of unsweetened muesli.
A cup of weak tea or herb tea.

Mid-morning: 6 dried apricots. A glass of fruit or vegetable juice.

Lunch: lettuce soup – soften half a chopped onion in a large pan with a little olive oil and add half a shredded Iceberg lettuce, stir for a couple of minutes, add 900ml/1½pints of vegetable stock and lots of black pepper, then simmer for 20 minutes before sprinkling with a large handful of chopped parsley. Enjoy with a chunk of crusty wholemeal bread with no butter.
A cup of herb or weak Indian tea.

Mid-afternoon: an apple and a pear.

Evening: pasta with lettuce pesto – use the rest of the Iceberg processed with a handful of pine nuts, a little olive oil, 1 clove of garlic and a carton of low-fat fromage frais. Tomato, onion and yellow pepper salad. Herb or weak Indian tea.

Treat your system gently on Day 4 and don't rush straight into your normal eating. It's best to avoid red meat and start with plainly cooked chicken or fish, some starchy foods and plenty of fruit, salads and vegetables. Don't eat dairy products apart from live yoghurt until Day 5.

This plan will stimulate your metabolism and almost certainly result in 1.5-2kg/3–4lb weight loss. Continue with any three days that you like to choose from my other diets. If necessary you can repeat the detox after two weeks, but you should not do it more than eight times a year and not more than twice in any three-month period.

EXCLUSION DIETS

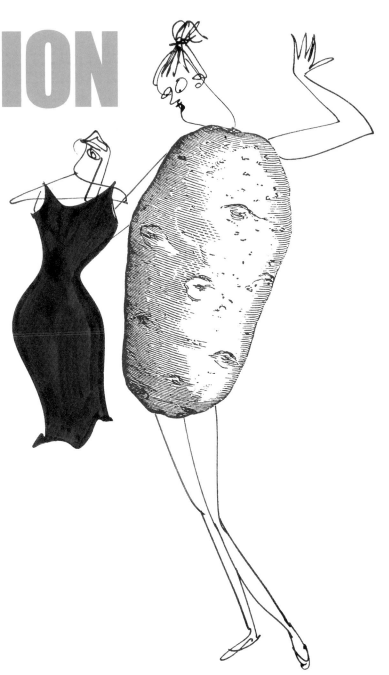

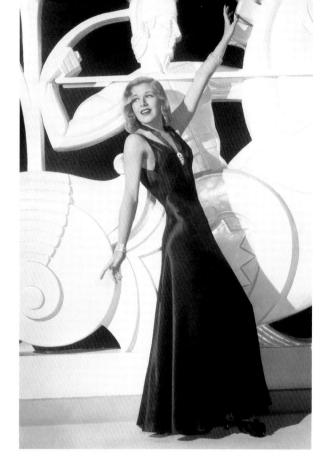

Many of you will have tried 101 different diets. You've starved on 1000 calories a day, struggled with meal replacements, eaten yourself silly on cabbage soup, cottage cheese, bananas, hard-boiled eggs and lettuce leaves without losing 500g/1lb at the end of it all. Scientific wisdom says that if you eat fewer calories than you burn up, the inevitable result is weightloss, but you've learned, in the words of the famous song: It ain't necessarily so. Why not? Of course, it's easy for your health advisor to sit behind a desk, wag an admonishing finger and say you've cheated. And it must be one of life's most frustrating experiences

when you've tried your utmost, stuck to the most minute detail of whatever diet you're following and finished just where you started – overweight. It's not generally accepted that food allergies or intolerances have any role to play in the success or failure of dietary regimes, but the most forward thinking of allergists – and naturopaths like me – have long recognised that there is a link between food allergies, the brain, behaviour and weight. People do have allergies to specific foods like shellfish, eggs, milk, nuts and strawberries, but most side effects after eating, especially those that happen between one and twenty-four hours later, are caused by food intolerance. Apart from milk, which is a common problem, other foods which may produce adverse effects include coffee, tea, cocoa, chocolate, cheese, beer, sausages, some canned foods, yeast, red wine, wheat and even tomatoes. Migraine, asthma, eczema, hives, irritable bowel syndrome, colitis, Crohn's disease, hayfever, rheumatoid-arthritis and menstrual problems are just some which may respond to dietary manipulation. If you have any of these problems and have found it virtually impossible to control your weight on any eating plan, the way your body reacts to some foods may lay at the heart of your difficulties. Unless food culprits are obvious, in which case you should avoid them, an exclusion diet is the best starting point. It might look difficult, but you only need to follow it rigorously for about two weeks, after which foods may be added back, provided you keep a record. You will soon be able to build a list of foods to which you are tolerant and eliminate the others. Stick rigidly to the diet for a fortnight and keep a diary to pinpoint bad reactions. After two weeks things should improve, but if not, food intolerance is probably not your problem so get further medical help. The following are the foods which you may and may not eat during the first two weeks of the exclusion diet:

	Not allowed	Allowed
Meat	preserved meats, bacon, sausages, all processed meat products	all other meats
Fish	smoked fish, shellfish	white fish
Vegetables	potatoes, onions, sweetcorn, aubergine (eggplant), sweet peppers, chillies, tomatoes	all other vegetables, salads, pulses, Swede(rutabaga) and parsnip
Fruit	citrus fruit e.g. oranges, grapefruit	all other fruit, e.g. apples, bananas, pears
Cereals	wheat, oats, barley, rye, corn	rice, ground rice, riceflakes, rice flour, sago, rice breakfast cereals, tapioca, millet, buckwheat, rice cakes
Cooking oils	corn oil, vegetable oil	sunflower oil, Soya oil, safflower oil, olive oil
Dairy products	cow's milk, butter, most margarines, cow's milk yoghurt them, dairy and trans fat-free margarines.	goat, sheep and Soya milk and products made from and cheese, eggs
Beverages	tea, coffee (beans, instant and decaffeinated),fruit squashes, orange juice, grapefruit juice, alcohol and tap water	herbal teas (e.g. camomile), fresh fruit juices(e.g. apple, pineapple), pure tomato juice (without additives), mineral, distilled or deionised water
Miscellaneous	chocolates, yeast, yeast extracts, artificial preservatives, colourings and flavourings, monosodium glutamate, all artificial sweeteners	carob, sea salt, herbs, spices, and small amounts of sugar or honey

After two weeks introduce other foods in this order: tap water, potatoes, cow's milk, yeast, tea, rye, butter, onions, eggs, porridge oats, coffee, chocolate, barley, citrus fruits, corn, cow's cheese, white wine, shellfish, natural cow's milk yoghurt, vinegar, wheat and nuts. Only try one new food every two days and if there is a reaction, don't try it again for at least a month. Carry on with the list when any symptoms stop. Any diet which is very restricted puts your health at risk and though it's alright to experiment on your own for a few weeks, any long term removal of major food groups should only be done under professional guidance.

THE
DESPERATION
DIET

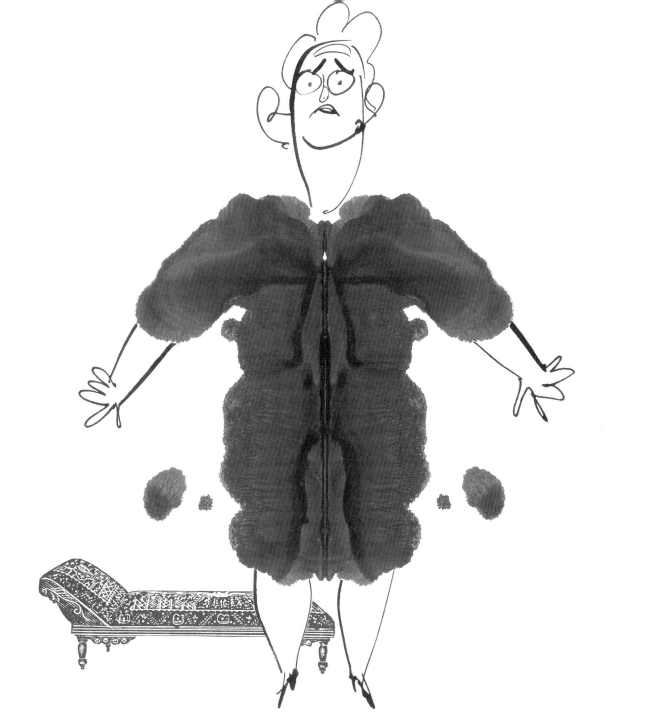

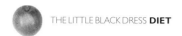

HOW TO LOSE 3.5KG/7LB IN 7 DAYS AND STILL EAT HEALTHILY

Many of you, including some of the men, will have tried at least a dozen different diets over the years, most of them in unsuccessful attempts at weight loss. And though nobody would deny that being seriously overweight is not good for your health, being a size 10 is not an automatic prescription for a life free of illness and disease.

Extreme starvation diets are unhealthy and never work, but when desperation is knocking at the door, you need desperate measures. You're going to a wedding, and you can't get into your new frock; your holiday's two weeks away and there are bulges hanging out of your bikini or love handles squeezing from your partner's trunks.

Then it's time for the Desperation Diet. For one week only and not more than three times a year, this is how to lose seven pounds in seven days without putting health at risk. This eating plan gives you a simple day-by-day list of menus, but by following the Wheel of Health guidelines, you can build a week's eating that suits your taste and lifestyle (page 21).

In the Desperation Diet there's no place for real treats like sweets, chocolates, cakes, biscuits, croissants and Danish pastries. If you're eating out, don't even look at the dessert menu. Put the evils of temptation behind you and just ask for some fresh fruit.

THE SEVEN-DAY DESPERATION DIET

At the beginning of each day add one measure of herbal Pure Plan (from health stores and chemists) to a litre bottle of still mineral water and make sure you drink it all by bedtime. This mixture of birch, meadowsweet and dandelion for fluid elimination, artichoke to stimulate the liver, burdock and wild pansy for the skin, fennel and fucus to stimulate metabolism, and tamarind and prune for the digestive system, will help you to that half stone weight loss by the end of the week.

Also, take 1 teaspoon of Swiss herbal tonic Bio-Strath before each meal and a daily Genesis vitamin and mineral pill with extra iron included.

DAY 1

Breakfast: half a grapefruit, 1 poached egg and 2 poached tomatoes.

Light meal: avocado, tomato and mushroom salad plus 125g/4oz low-fat cottage cheese and a large bunch of grapes.

Main meal: a large bowl of thinly sliced cucumber with lots of black pepper, cider vinegar and a teaspoon of extra virgin olive oil, a good portion of stir-fried vegetables served on a bed of plain boiled rice.

DAY 2

Breakfast: a large fresh peach and 6 ripe strawberries.

Light meal: a large green salad and a mixture of lot of steamed vegetables – carrots, courgettes, new potatoes, peas, runner beans, sweet corn – tossed in a mean teaspoon of butter and sprinkled with fresh chopped mint and parsley.

Main meal: a bowl of vegetable soup, a large red or yellow pepper stuffed with rice, and a generous portion of lightly-cooked spinach chopped with a drizzle of virgin olive oil and a clove of crushed garlic.

DAY 3

Breakfast: a large bowl of cherries and a low-fat live yoghurt.

Light meal: mixed green salad and a generous portion of your favourite pasta drizzled with olive oil, crushed garlic, sprinkled with fresh chopped parsley.

Main meal: a carton of low-fat live yoghurt mixed with chopped cucumber, lots of fresh mint, garlic, black pepper, a teaspoon of extra virgin olive oil. Skinless grilled chicken breast, with grilled tomato, iceberg lettuce and boiled or baked potatoes.

DAY 4

Breakfast: muesli, porridge, Shredded wheat, Weetabix or other wholegrain cereal, with semi-skimmed milk, and a banana.

Light meal: a sliced hard-boiled egg with chunks of tomato, cucumber, fennel and lettuce in wholemeal pita bread.

Main meal: Celery, apple and walnut salad, grilled trout with cauliflower and runner beans tossed in a teaspoon of olive oil and a squeeze of lemon juice, sprinkled with lots of parsley.

DAY 5

Breakfast: large bunch of grapes.

Light meal: crudités of olives, radishes, carrot, fennel and celery, any vegetable soup, a wholewheat roll and a pear.

Main meal: generous portion of mixed curried vegetables, served on plain boiled rice. A tomato and onion salad.

DAY 6

Breakfast: mixed summer fruits.

Light meal: a large tomato stuffed with mixed tuna and low fat cottage cheese, plenty of black pepper and a green salad.

Main meal: Stir-fried cubes of chicken, beef, lamb or tofu, with mixed stir-fried vegetables and noodles. Mixed fresh berries with low-fat live yoghurt flavoured with the zest of a lemon, quarter of a teaspoon of cinnamon, a teaspoon of honey and 2 fresh mint leaves.

DAY 7

Breakfast: a boiled egg and 1 slice of wholemeal toast very thinly scraped with butter, a glass of fresh unsweetened juice.

Light meal: salad of red radicchio and chicory leaves with grilled mushrooms and a wholemeal roll, an apple and a pear.

Main meal: a salad of pink grapefruit and peach with low-fat fromage frais, grilled salmon steak with boiled potatoes and a green vegetable, a matchbox-sized portion of low-fat cheese with a stick of celery

All week make sure you drink 1 litre/1½ pints water plus Pure Plan, and the same again of other drinks – herb tea, unsweetened or unsalted fruit and vegetable juice, weak tea. By the end of this week your desperation will turn to delight. Seven pounds lighter in seven days, clear skin, bright eyes and bursting with energy. Your reward for sticking to the Desperation Diet! Now keep your weight off and stay well with the Wheel of Health as your guide (page 21).

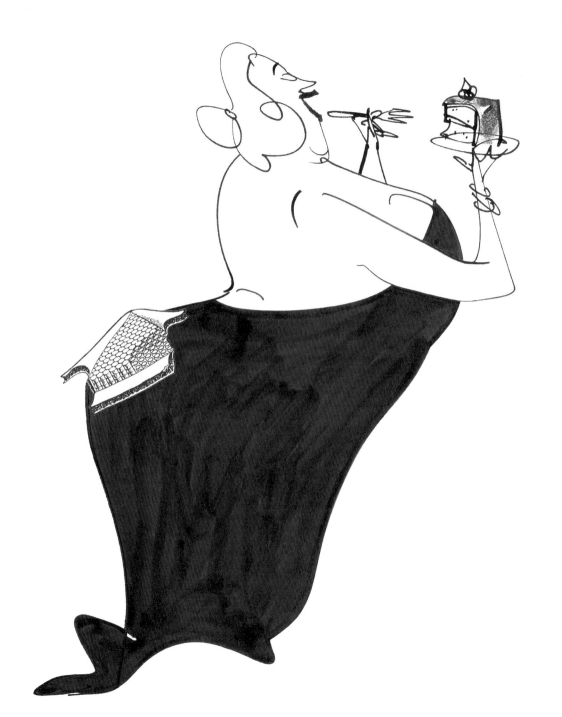

FOOD COMBINING

Dr. William Howard Hay was one of the great pioneers of the food reform movement. After suffering severe ill health himself and getting no relief from his doctors in America at the turn of the century, he decided to take matters into his own hands and to treat his condition by making radical changes to his diet. He decided to eat only such things as he believed were intended by nature as food for man, taking them in natural form and in quantities no greater than seemed necessary for his present need. This return to fundamental eating produced dramatic changes in his health, and after three months he had returned to his former vigour. He then applied the same principles to treating his own patients and finally in his book, 'A New Health Era', outlined the principles of the Hay system of eating.

Before the First World War Hay suggested that the over-consumption of white flour products, refined sugar and other refined carbohydrates, the eating of too much meat, and constipation were vital factors in the cause of many digestive disorders and other health complaints. How interesting that the most up-to-date thinking on nutrition and health implicates many of the same factors.

The fundamental principle of the Hay diet is that starch foods and protein foods are not eaten at the same time – no bread and cheese, fish and chips, or meat and potatoes. He divided foods into protein, neutral and starch and allowed his patients to eat neutral foods with starch or protein, but always with a gap of at least four hours between eating foods of different groups. In recent years the Hay diet has become a popular 'cure-all' for every conceivable ailment and its success attributed to a variety of pseudoscientific theories.

In practice I have found it unnecessary to apply all Hay's rules too rigidly and I certainly don't recommend food combining as The Way of Eating for Life. Sticking to the food combining rules certainly has a dramatic effect on the treatment of people with a wide variety of digestive problems, especially chronic indigestion with no obvious cause. I've no idea how or why it works, but it does. What's more,

there's a bonus, if you're overweight, following the Hay diet will help you shed a few surplus pounds. I'm sure that the discipline of sticking to the rules of food combining and the amount of time needed to shop, plan and prepare the food, means that people eat in a much healthier way.

Try it for yourself and see how simple it is after a little practice. After all, you don't have to give up anything, you just have to eat in a different way. The following list will give you an idea of where various foods should go in the scheme, and the one week menu will help with your own planning. Eat one starch meal, one protein meal and one meal of mostly fruits, vegetables and salads each day. Try to leave four hours between starch and protein meals, but if you have to nibble, try to stick to the neutral food list.

Protein	Neutral	Starch
Meat	All vegetables except potatoes	Potatoes
Poultry	All nuts except peanuts	Bread
Game	Butter	Flour, oats, wheat, barley
Fish	Cream	Rice
Shellfish	Egg yolks	Millet
Whole eggs	Sesame, sunflower and olive oils	Rye
Cheese, milk and yoghurt	All salads	Buckwheat
All fruits, except those in the starch group	Seeds and sprouted seeds	Bananas, pears, papayas, grapes
All the legumes – lentils, dried beans	Herbs	Dried fruits
Red wine	Honey	Yoghurt
Dry white wine	Maple syrup	Beer
	Gin and whisky	

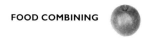

MONDAY

Breakfast: Sliced blood oranges and pink grapefruit. A helping of creamy yoghurt, with nuts and honey if liked.

Light meal or snack: Scrambled Eggs with Mushrooms (page 61). Tossed salad. Breakfast Compôte (page 63 – make enough for 2 meals)

Main meal: Stuffed Peppers with Rice. Peas. Sticks of celery. Dates and figs.

TUESDAY

Breakfast: Breakfast Compôte (page 63). An orange. Yoghurt.

Light meal or snack: Gratin of mushrooms and potatoes. Lettuce and watercress salad. A ripe sweet pear.

Main meal: Mustard-marinated salmon. Spinach purée with nutmeg. Stewed apricots with almonds and honey.

WEDNESDAY

Breakfast: Hot wholewheat rolls with butter. A banana.

Light meal or snack: Risotto with finely chopped tomatoes, spring onions, celery and red pepper. Tossed green salad. Raisins and nuts.

Main meal: Aubergine puree with crudites – raw carrot, celery, cucumber, fennel, sprigs of cauliflower, to dip in. Meat balls in tomato sauce. Green beans. Sticks of celery.

THURSDAY

Breakfast: An orange. Half a pink grapefruit. Yoghurt, honey and nuts.

Light meal or snack: Baked potato with butter or sour cream, and plenty of chopped fresh herbs. Finely chopped red pepper, tomato and cucumber salad served on lettuce leaves. A ripe sweet pear.

Main meal: Grilled steak, chops or cutlets. Cabbage and carrots. Breakfast Compôte (page 63 – make enough for 2 meals).

FRIDAY

Breakfast: Breakfast Compôte with yoghurt, or a little single cream.

Light meal or snack: Half an avocado pear, sliced, with cress, tomatoes, cucumber, on lettuce with a little oil and a drop or two of lemon dressing. Crusty wholewheat roll and a little butter.

Main meal: Beetroot and apple soup (any vegetable soup but no rice or pasta). Grilled, steamed, baked fish – your own favourite recipe. Steamed broccoli and courgettes (zucchini).

SATURDAY

Breakfast: An orange. An apple. A banana. Yoghurt.

Light meal or snack: Salad Niçoise. Sticks of celery. Rye crispbread with a little cream cheese.

Main meal: Chicken and Vegetable Stir-Fry with spinach or chard. A tossed green salad. Stewed or baked apple with cinnamon and cloves.

SUNDAY

Breakfast: Orange or grapefruit juice. A selection of tropical fruits. Yoghurt.

Light meal or snack: Bruschetta made with a slice of thick coarse bread, toasted, rubbed with garlic, covered in strips of red and yellow peppers, sundried tomatoes, a drizzle of olive oil and cooked under a very hot grill for a couple of minutes. Cucumber, lettuce and watercress salad.

Main meal: Crudités. Any roast or grilled meat with squash, broccoli and leeks. Crème Brûlée, crème caramel or ice cream.

Use these menus as a guide to preparing your own favourite dishes. You'll soon get used to this different way of eating, which is not as difficult as it seems once you've had a little practice.

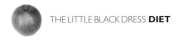

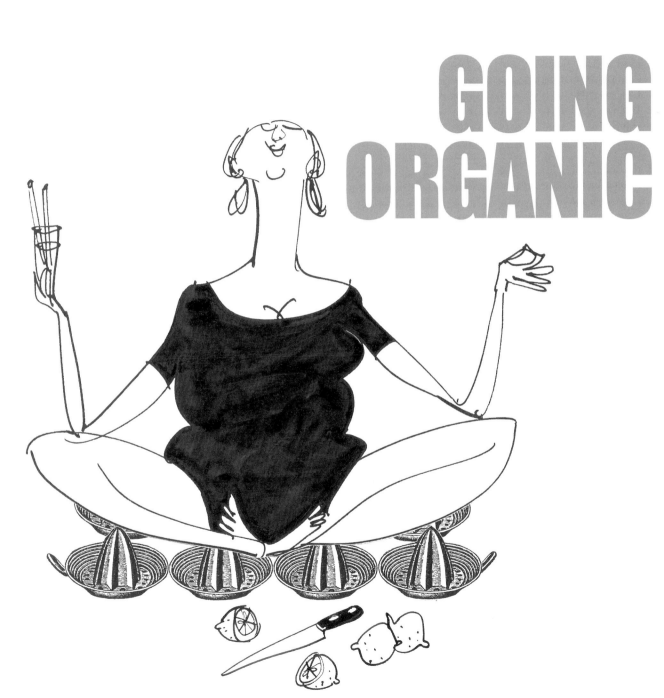

GOING ORGANIC

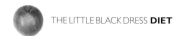

WANT TO BE A HEALTHY SLIMMER? GO ORGANIC

Is organic food better for you if you're dieting? The answer has to be a resounding 'yes', and that's true whether you're trying to lose weight or not. It's better for the consumer, better for the producer and better for the environment that we all have to live in. If you're reducing the total quantity of food you eat, it becomes even more important that what you do consume is food of the highest nutritional quality. And there is now overwhelming evidence that organically grown produce is now richer in many of the essential nutrients like vitamins and minerals than their non-organic equivalents.

Good quality organic produce is not only free of all the hazardous agricultural chemicals but if you're buying manufactured goods there's an added bonus. They are made without the use of artificial colourings, flavourings, preservatives or any other of the thousands of synthetic substances used in the food processing industry. This becomes even more important when you're doing cleansing or eliminating diets as you lower the overall toxic load that your body has to process and eliminate.

You don't have to take my word for it – a report from The Soil Association, the world's leading organic organisation, says there is now irrefutable evidence that organically grown crops are not only chemical-free but also have higher levels of essential nutrients than non-organic equivalents. After analysing more than 400 published studies Patrick Holden, Director of the Association, says they found that organic crops have more vitamin C and essential minerals and they're also richer in phytonutrients than those on which chemicals are used.

Phytonutrients form a vital group of natural plant chemicals which help to protect growing crops from damaging insects, fungal infections and viruses. They're also known to be a major part of the human body's own defences against cell damage and many forms of cancer. The Government's figures reveal that almost 90 per cent of women between the ages of 19 and 50 get less iron from their food than their minimum daily requirement; the daily need for selenium – a mineral vital for a healthy heart and protection against breast and prostate cancer – is 70 micrograms, yet the daily consumption is now often only as low as 30 micrograms.

As the march of intensive factory farming has spread across the countryside, official Government tables show a frightening decline in the levels of essential minerals in our everyday foods over the last 50 years. Broccoli, carrots, tomatoes and strawberries have lost around half or more of their calcium; spinach, swedes, carrots and apples now contain 60 per cent less iron; potassium and magnesium in watercress, runner beans, potatoes, green peppers and carrots have fallen by 30-75 per cent. So is it any wonder that more people are beginning to turn to naturally grown, properly fertilised and nutrient-rich organic foods?

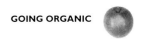

PERCENTAGE NUTRIENT LOSS OVER 50 YEARS

	Calcium	Iron	Potassium	Magnesium	Selenium
Broccoli	75				
Carrots	45	50	23	75	
Tomatoes	50		14	37	
Strawberries		55			
Raspberries		39			
Blackberries		35			
Spring onions		74			
Spinach		60			
Swede		70			
Watercress	23		26	12	
Apples		66			
Oranges		66	25		
Green peppers				43	
Runner beans				21	30
Potatoes			37	29	
Whiteflour					43
Wholemeal bread					52
Melons				45	

The amount of chemicals used in conventional non-organic production of fruit and vegetables is horrendous. The average lettuce may be sprayed 11 times during its short growing life, apple and pear trees are sprayed to slow down ripening and stick fruit on the trees when prices are low, or speed it up when there's a shortage and prices rise. Fruit is treated with wax to extend its shelf life and citrus fruits heavily covered in fungicides as well as wax – make sure you only use organic, or at least unwaxed lemons, to add to your early morning hot water. Each year over 25,000 tons of the 500 different licensed pesticides are sprayed onto the food you eat.

The contamination of mothers' milk with chemicals and antibiotics used in farming also presents a hazard to the health of babies. During pre-conceptual planning, pregnancy, breast-feeding, infancy and early childhood the importance of organic foods is paramount. So much so that one of the UK's leading foetal and infant toxicology experts has gone public on this issue. In a report 'What are babies eating?' Dr. Vyvyan Howard at the University of Liverpool says, 'One of the most positive things we can do is eat organic food. This considerably reduces the "body burden" of toxic chemicals in both parent and child. Organic food in its many forms avoids all the possible exposures to pesticides during growing, harvesting and storing food before you eat it.'

Anyone concerned about their weight and trying to shed a little must understand the great significance of switching from non-organic to organic meat and dairy products. This simple change can make a fundamental difference to helping your body get rid of unwanted and unhealthy fat. When it comes to free-range animals, there is a dramatic difference in the quality of both meat and milk. Not only does free-range beef contain less saturated fat when compared with intensively reared livestock, but it contains far higher levels of a naturally occurring fatty acid called Conjugated Linoleic Acid (CLA). CLA is essential to the way in which the body uses and stores fat from your diet but most people don't get enough of it from their food.

American Professor Mike Pariza isolated CLA from free-range beef and found that it was anti-carcinogenic. He's been researching the properties of this special fatty acid for years and found that it's also a key factor in weight management, as it helps reduce total body fat and increase muscle tone. Unfortunately the vast majority of cattle are not free-range any more, so the content of CLA in both meat and dairy products has declined dramatically. Unless you choose organic varieties you're unlikely to get as much as you need.

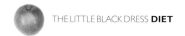

As the organic movement grows, an increasing number of 'experts' appear on radio, TV and in your daily papers trying to warn about the dangers of organic food, particularly stories about the risks of bacterial contamination from farmyard manure. The factory farming lobby and the Food Standards Agency are at pains to point out that the use of all these chemicals is strictly controlled and the amounts that get into our food are negligible – well they would say that wouldn't they?

Nothing could be further from the truth. Recent examination of 3,000 samples of fresh organic produce failed to find one instance of bacterial contamination – no-one uses fresh animal manure as it would kill most plants. It's usually composted for at least 12 months and the heat generated kills the bugs. Conversely, 56 per cent of lettuces randomly analysed by Government scientists were found to have higher pesticide residues than the maximum allowed, 42 per cent had multiple residues that exceeded the limits and one sample contained an agricultural chemical prohibited in the UK.

A Europe-wide study found illegal synthetic hormones in steaks and liver purchased throughout the Community. Spain and Belgium were the worst offenders with the highest levels of these extremely dangerous chemicals, with Holland, Germany and the UK not far behind. Denmark appears to be the only country not illegally using growth hormones. Organic meat is the only really safe option and if you're going to America, don't eat meat at all – growth hormones are legally permitted in the USA.

Of course we can't all go totally organic overnight, though what a wonderful thing that would be for the health of the nation and of the planet. Even though organic food has come down considerably in price and some locally grown organic produce at the height of its season is often cheaper than the supermarket, cost is an important factor. For most of us it's a question of making the right choices. This list may help you decide what to do.

FIVE ESSENTIAL ORGANICS TO HELP YOUR WEIGHT LOSS PROGRAMME

These are foods which most families consume consistently and in quite substantial quantities. Enjoy the flavour, reduce the risk and choose:-

1 Milk; any family with children should put this at the top of the list. It's a little more expensive but for a family of 4 drinking 1.5litres/2 pints a day it's less than the price of a second class stamp.

2 Yoghurt, butter, cheese and other dairy products; organic butter used modestly is much better for your health than any margarine – but yoghurts and cheese may cost a little more. Worth it to avoid antibiotics and the fat soluble toxic chemicals.

3 Eggs and poultry; this will cost a bit more but the real difference in flavour certainly makes it worthwhile, as well as the reduced risk of salmonella, antibiotics and chemical residue from intensive feed.

4 Bread and flour; apart from being free from chemicals used when the wheat is growing, you'll avoid the food chemicals added during baking and processing. An organic wholemeal loaf costs more but try baking your own. Buy Canadian organic bread-making flour and you'll get masses of selenium which we're so short of in the UK.

5 Carrots, potatoes and other root vegetables; even the Government has issued warnings to remove the tops, bottoms and peel from non-organic carrots. Root vegetables absorb and concentrate chemicals including harmful nitrates, fungicides and pesticides.

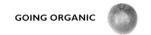

FIVE ORGANIC LUXURIES WHICH WON'T MAKE MUCH DIFFERENCE TO YOUR WEIGHT LOSS

1 Tea and coffee; while both these crops are heavily sprayed, very little residue remains after roasting, drying and fermenting. The main benefit of choosing organic versions is that it protects the plantation workers from unacceptable exposure to the dangerous chemicals.

2 Organic wine, beer and spirits; you shouldn't be drinking too much of these anyway and organic wine is frequently a misleading label. Even if the grapes are grown organically this doesn't mean that chemical additives are not used during the winemaking process. Drink real ale or buy imported German beers where it's forbidden to add chemicals of any sort.

3 Cola drinks, fruit drinks and squashes; organic brands are a cynical marketing exercise to persuade you to spend more money on junk drinks for your kids. A can of organic cola still contains around 8 teaspoons of sugar which is no good for your children whether it's organic or not.

4 Organic exotic fruit; unless you're eating 4 mangoes, 2 pineapples and a dozen kiwi fruit a week, this is going to cost you a lot more money for very little benefit. In any case apart from the health benefits a prime objective of the organic movement is to reduce 'food miles' – the organic pineapple will travel several thousand adding to pollution, global warming and energy costs.

5 Organic spices; these are considerably more expensive and how much chemical residue are you going to get from 3 peppercorns, 1 clove or a pinch of cinnamon. If money doesn't matter they're fine but, for the vast majority of us, put them at the bottom of your priority list.

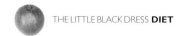

RECIPES

**All recipes are for 4 people
unless otherwise stated**

HEALTHY BREAKFAST IDEAS

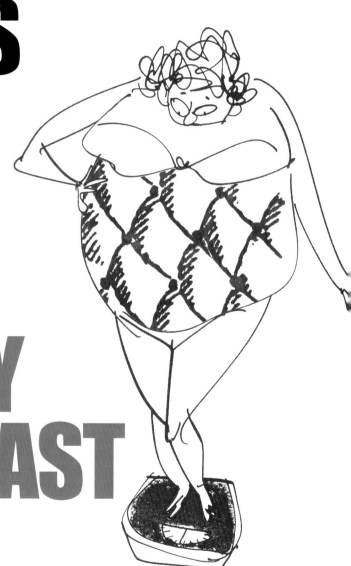

If you wake up at 6.30, jump into the shower and have to catch a train or be on the road within an hour, it's very tempting to think: 'Breakfast? Forget it.' If you're also trying to lose weight, you may feel that's a good way to start the day; if I don't have breakfast, I won't want much lunch, but I can eat what I want when I'm more relaxed in the evening.

This simply isn't true. The old adage that you should breakfast like a king, lunch like a prince and dine like a pauper really is the best nutritional advice.

Your body needs that boost of energy in the morning to set you up for the physical – and mental – demands of the day. Arrive at work or get home after taking the kids to school with your blood sugar levels sliding and stress levels heading up the wall and you'll almost certainly reach for the nearest quick-fix snack – a high-calorie Danish from the office canteen or one of the chocolate bars you bought specially as a treat for the kids.

You'll feel great for about half an hour, then your blood sugar level will plummet and you'll want more. You'll be into a very vicious nutritional circle for the rest of the day.

Most of us don't have much time to spend preparing breakfast – and you really don't have to. Here are some simple, nutritious starts to the day

• A cup of hot water mixed with soya milk and 2 tablespoons of molasses.

• Stewed apples sprinkled with flaked almonds – you can make three days' worth of apples and keep them in the fridge.

• Baked beans on toast with a grilled tomato.

• Porridge made with half water and semi-skimmed milk. A slice of wholemeal toast with a little butter and honey.

• Half a grapefruit, 2 poached eggs, 2 grilled tomatoes.

• An orange, an apple and a pear sliced into a bowl of natural yoghurt and topped with a teaspoon of honey.

• 2 boiled eggs and 2 slices of wholemeal toast spread thinly with butter.

• 2 slices of wholemeal toast spread with organic peanut butter and a sliced banana on top.

At weekends, when you may have more time, you can make more of a meal of breakfast. I love a lie-in on Sunday mornings and to wake up to something special and listen to The Archers. Some of my favourites are on the next page:

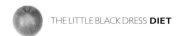

SUPERBRUNCH

Smoked salmon and eggs is a traditional, almost clichéd, brunch combination. But, if you add spinach for its cancer-protective phytochemicals, and almonds for good protein, zinc and selenium, you'll have a really good start to your day of leisure. These quantities are enough for two people.

75g/2³/₄oz unsalted butter
100ml/3¹/₂floz milk
5 organic eggs
125g/4¹/₄oz smoked salmon cut in small pieces – buy
  the off-cuts from a good fishmonger if possible
450g/1lb fresh baby spinach leaves
1 tablespoon extra virgin olive oil
1 tablespoon roasted, unsalted, chopped almonds
1 tablespoon chopped parsley

• Add the butter and milk to a deep frying pan
• Break in the eggs and scramble
• After 2 or 3 minutes add the smoked salmon
• Wash the spinach, put in a saucepan without adding water, cover and cook till soft
• Strain, add the olive oil and nuts and chop finely
• Serve the scrambled egg on top of the spinach and sprinkle with parsley

REAL SWISS MUESLI

Proper muesli isn't just something you just pour out of a packet and drown in milk in the morning. To do it properly – as they do at the Bircher-Benner Clinic in Switzerland, where this breakfast dish was first created – you need to start the night before. These quantities are for one person – just double or triple them where necessary but make sure the dish you use is large enough to allow the muesli to expand to about twice the size of the original ingredients.

3 tablespoons organic, unsweetened muesli
1 dessertspoonful seedless raisins
2 tablespoons low-fat, bio-natural yoghurt
half a glass of fruit juice – apple, orange or pineapple. It's
  best to make it yourself, but freshly-squeezed from the
  supermarket will do
1 apple
1 pear
2 teaspoons runny honey

• Put the muesli, raisins and yoghurt into a bowl and add the juice
• Leave in the fridge overnight
• In the morning, peel and grate the apple and pear
• Add to the muesli mixture and drizzle with the honey

You can add any type of fruit to this muesli mixture . . . sliced bananas, ready-to-eat dried exotic fruit – it's easier to snip them with a pair of scissors than make more washing up by chopping them on a board – sliced strawberries, whole raspberries or blueberries. The world is your fruit bowl.

SCRAMBLED EGGS WITH MUSHROOMS

Eggs have had a bad press in recent years. Salmonella and cholesterol are just two of the reasons which have made people turn their back on this inexpensive, nourishing and delicious food. Eggs do contain cholesterol, but they aren't the reason your arteries get clogged with this fatty substance. That's caused by the cholesterol your body makes when you eat too much saturated animal fat. To avoid salmonella, buy organic and free-range eggs.

These quantities are enough for two people. You can halve the quantities to make it for one, but don't make more than this amount in one batch because the eggs will overcook.

50g/1½oz butter
100g/4oz chestnut mushrooms
6 medium organic eggs
1 tablespoon parsley, chopped

- Melt the butter gently in a non-stick but quite deep frying pan
- Wipe, but don't wash, the mushrooms and simmer them, covered, over a very gentle heat for 10 minutes
- Meanwhile, whisk the eggs coarsely, leaving some of the white and yolk separated
- Add to the mushroom and butter in the pan
- Keeping the heat very low, leave until the eggs just start to become solid
- Push the egg gently in from the sides without breaking up the whites and yolks too much
- Continue cooking until you think they're nearly done, then remove from the heat. They'll finish very well on their own in the hot pan for about a minute
- Chop the parsley, sprinkle it on top and serve on toast

You can also prepare this recipe in exactly the same way using coarsely chopped tomatoes or a mixture of mushrooms and tomatoes, but keep to the proportion of vegetables to eggs mentioned above or the whole dish will be far too watery.

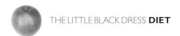

ANTOINETTA'S ITALIAN BREAKFAST

Some of the best recipes I've collected are from my patients, especially those who come from other countries – Spain, France, Africa, Asia, Greece, the West Indies and the Middle East. I'm also extremely lucky to have a wonderful Italian hairdresser who comes to my house and lets me fall asleep while she trims my beard. Carmela is Italian and loves to cook, so when I do manage to stay awake we talk endlessly about food. This is one of her mother's favourite dishes.

450g/1lb new potatoes

2 largish courgettes

1 medium onion

olive oil

coarse sea salt

black pepper

4 organic, free-range eggs

4 sprigs of mint

- Scrub, but don't peel, the potatoes
- Slice them thinly
- Wash, but don't peel, the courgettes
- Slice them thinly
- Peel and chop the onion
- Thinly cover a large frying pan with the olive oil
- Gently sweat the onions until soft
- Layer the potatoes on top of the onions
- Sprinkle with a tiny amount of salt
- After a minute or two, turn the potatoes, mix with the onions and cook until they start to go soft, adding a little extra oil if necessary
- Layer the courgettes on top of the potato mix and season generously with black pepper
- Turn up the heat a little and continue to cook, turning gently and making sure that the vegetables don't break up
- When the courgettes are almost done, add the eggs, 1 to each corner of the pan, and use a fork to break the yolks and pull them gently across the mixture. They shouldn't look like scrambled eggs
- Leave the pan on a moderate heat until the eggs are set – about 2 minutes
- Serve each portion with a sprig of mint

Don't worry if you think you've made too much – this dish is just as delicious cold. It's a great slimmer's breakfast, providing protein, vitamins and minerals and loads of energy to keep you going until lunchtime.

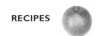

BREAKFAST COMPOTE

Fruit is a wonderful way to start the day and get your digestive system up and running – essential when you don't want to pile on the weight. Yes, you do have to start the night before, but you can make three days' supply of this delicious breakfast and keep it in the fridge.

dried apricots

dried prunes

dried figs

dried any other fruits that are available

fresh apple juice

cinnamon

at least 1 lemon

natural, live bio-yoghurt

• Put the fruit into a dish

• Cover with boiling water

• Wait until the water has cooled and top up with apple juice so that all the fruit is covered

• Add the cinnamon – 1 pinch for every 450g/1lb of fruit – and mix in gently

• Slice the lemon and float on top

• Leave in the fridge overnight

• Serve with a dollop of yoghurt on top

TOMMY OMMY

You have to be very lucky to get a decent omelette when you eat out – they're normally over-cooked and rubbery because of the paranoia about runny eggs and salmonella. Buy organic, free-range eggs from a salmonella-free flock and you won't have this concern. My wife, Sally, is the omelette queen in our home and this is the fool-proof way to make the best tomato omelette you've ever tasted. There's no alternative to butter for a good omelette, but Sally's method keeps it to a minimum. These quantities are for two people, but they need to be cooked separately.

50g/1½oz unsalted butter

4 large organic tomatoes

1 teaspoon dried oregano or half a handful of fresh, chopped leaves

5 large organic and free-range eggs

black pepper

• Melt the butter gently in a non-stick frying or omelette pan

• Chop the tomatoes and add to the pan

• If you're using dried oregano, add it now

• Cook the tomatoes gently for about 2 minutes

• Whisk the eggs in a jug

• Remove the tomatoes, but leave the butter in the pan

• Add half of the egg mixture and cook gently for 1 minute, until just holding its shape

• Pour on half the tomatoes and, if using fresh oregano, half the leaves

• Continue cooking until nearly done, then remove and allow to finish with the residue heat in the pan

• Using a wooden palette, fold in half and season with black pepper

• Repeat with the remaining eggs

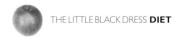

GRILLED PINEAPPLES

Fresh pineapple is the perfect way to start your day. It's very low in calories and rich in the natural enzyme bromelain, which is a powerful digestive aid. I was first served this at one of the most exciting Indian restaurants in London, Chor Bazar, as a dessert – then cooked it the following morning. Adding cinnamon gives the dish even more digestive benefits.

pineapple
cinnamon
1 tablespoon demerara sugar
1 heaped teaspoon ground cinnamon
125g/4¹/₂oz blueberries, raspberries or any small berries
    available

• Peel, core and slice the pineapple into rings
• Place the slices on a sheet of foil on a grill pan
• Mix the cinnamon and sugar thoroughly and sprinkle on each pineapple ring
• Place under a hot grill until the sugar melts and starts to bubble – about 3 minutes
• Serve with the fresh berries in the centre of the pineapple

Over the years I've learned to stop buying endless kitchen gadgets. Most of them are no use and just end up gathering dust in the drawers. But there's always an exception to the rule and The Pineapple Corer and Peeler made by VACU-VIN is cheap, simple and really works.

TOFU TORTILLA

Rich in calcium and plant oestrogens, this is a high-protein women's breakfast. I always think it's a great shame that tofu is regarded only as food for vegetarians as its all-rouhd health benefits should be enjoyed by everyone. This power breakfast is full of betacarotenes, vitatims A and C and the legendary healthy properties of garlic. Not a recipe when you're rushing off to work, but ideal for those lovely lazy Sunday mornings.

1 small onion
1 clove garlic
1 tablespoon extra virgin olive oil
1 teaspoon turmeric
1 teaspoon cumin
half each of a red and yellow pepper
1 small tin of sweetcorn
1 tablespoon chopped coriander leaves
450g/1lb tofu
1 teaspoon light soy sauce
4 wholewheat tortillas
4 tablespoons spicy tomato salsa

• Sweat the onions and garlic in the olive oil
• When soft, add the turmeric and cumin and stir for 1 minute
• Desseed and chop the peppers and add them to the pan
• Continue cooking until they're soft
• Add the drained sweetcorn and chopped coriander and crumble in the tofu
• Stir in the soya sauce and cook for another 4 minutes
• Spoon the mixture onto the tortillas
• Roll them up and serve each 1 with a dollop of salsa

Marilyn Monroe, Jack Lemmon and Tony Curtis in
Some Like It Hot, 1959

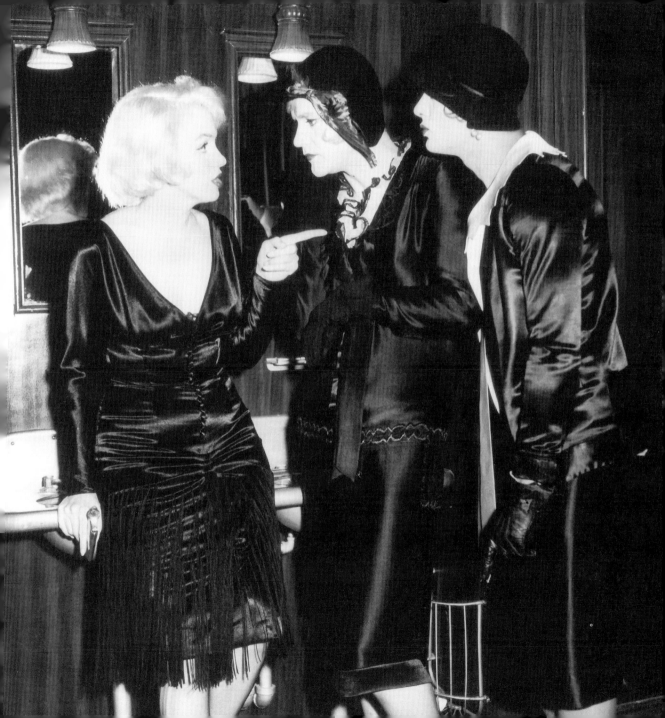

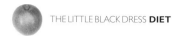

MAIN MEALS

PM PASTA

An ideal recipe for women with difficult periods; it contains lots of starch, which keeps you on an even keel and copes with mood swings, as well as oily fish for essential fatty acids. It's also rich in minerals, especially calcium, zinc and iron.

400g/14oz wholemeal fusilli

4 tablespoon olive oil

3 chopped cloves garlic

8 spring onions, sliced finely lengthways

2 tablespoons cashew nuts

2 tablespoons pumpkin seeds

1 x 400g/14oz tin of salmon, drained and flaked

225g/8oz tofu, diced

black pepper, freshly ground

- Cook the pasta according to the instructions on the packet
- While it's cooking, heat the oil in a pan and gently sweat the garlic
- When the garlic is soft, add the spring onions, nuts and seeds
- After 2 minutes, add the salmon and tofu
- Put cooked pasta into a warmed bowl
- Add the warmed salmon mixture
- Season with black pepper and mix thoroughly

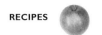

ITALIAN STEAK IN RED WINE

As long as your family are carnivores, this is a really quick meal and tastes great with baby new potatoes for mopping up the sauce. The dish is full of protein, iron and has the protective value of red wine.

2 tablespoon rapeseed oil
25g/1oz unsalted butter
4 tablespoons plain flour
4 fillet steaks, cut about 2.5cm/1in thick
2 cloves garlic, crushed
300ml/10fl oz decent **Chianti** or **Barolo**
black pepper, freshly ground

• Heat the oil and butter in a large pan
• Put the flour on a plate and coat the steaks
• Add them to the pan with the garlic, cook on each side for 1 minute and remove with a slotted spoon
• Add the wine and turn up the heat, stirring constantly to loosen the bits stuck to the bottom of the pan, until most of the wine has evaporated
• Season the steaks with black pepper, return to the pan and cook each side for 2 or 3 minutes, depending on how rare you want them

CHICKEN AND VEGETABLE STIR FRY

This high-protein, low-fat meal is full of vitamins and flavour and it can be ready in as long as it takes to cook the rice.

225g/8oz rice
2 tablespoons rapeseed oil
2 garlic cloves, crushed
6 thin slices ginger root, optional
4 chicken breasts
1 large pack fresh stir-fry vegetables
2 teaspoons sesame seeds
4 teaspoons soya sauce

• Boil the rice and, when it is almost cooked, heat the oil in a wok or large frying pan
• Add the garlic, ginger and chicken, stirring vigorously for 2 minutes, or until the meat is browned all over
• Add the vegetables, sesame seeds and soya sauce, stirring until the vegetables are cooked, about 5 minutes
• Drain the rice and put it in the centre of a large plate, with chicken and vegetables in the middle

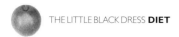
COURGETTE PASTA

Pasta has to be one of the healthiest foods around. A complex carbohydrate, it's packed with slow-release energy, as well as some protein and minerals. This recipe really couldn't be simpler and it's perfect diet food.

400g/14oz of your favourite pasta
3 courgettes, finely grated
50g/2oz unsalted butter
black pepper, freshly ground
2 tablespoons Parmesan cheese, grated

- Cook pasta according to the instructions on the packet
- Drain and stir in the uncooked courgettes immediately, as the heat from the pasta will soften them
- Add in the butter, season with black pepper.
- Sprinkle on the Parmesan and serve

MACKIE BURGERS

Don't worry about the little bit of butter and, whatever you do, don't use margarine. Made in a factory, not on a farm, margarine contains harmful trans-fats. Oily fish provides essential fatty acids, which are good for the brain, heart and joints. Keep these fish burgers covered in the fridge if you want to eat them cold.

500g/18oz cooked or canned mackerel fillets
350g/12oz mashed potato
50g/2oz butter
6 spring onions, chopped
2 tablespoons chopped parsley
2 tablespoons vegetable stock or milk
2 tablespoons fine oatmeal
rapeseed oil, for frying

- Flake the mackerel
- Mix with the mashed potato, melted butter, spring onions and parsley
- If mixture is very stiff, moisten with a little stock or milk
- Shape into burgers and chill for half an hour
- Dust with oatmeal and fry in the oil in a pan on both sides until golden brown
- Drain on kitchen paper

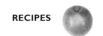

SWEET STUFFED PEPPERS

These very different vegetarian peppers are wonderful hot or cold. They're very sustaining as they provide slow-release energy and they're bursting with essential betacarotene and B vitamins.

4 large red, yellow, orange or green peppers, or 1 of each
175g/6oz long-grain brown rice
400ml/14fl oz water
1 medium onion, peeled and sliced
1 large finely, grated carrot
2 tablespoons extra virgin olive oil
1 tablespoon pine nuts
1 tablespoon sunflower seeds
1 tablespoon raisins
1 tablespoon chopped fresh parsley
1 tablespoon finely chopped mint
black pepper, freshly ground

- Preheat the oven to 190°C/375°F/gas 5
- Wash peppers, slice off the stalk ends and keep as lids
- Carefully scoop out the fleshy ribs and seeds
- Wash the rice, put in a heavy pan with the water, bring to the boil, cover and simmer for 20 minutes
- Fry the onions and carrots in 1 tablespoon of oil until soft
- Add pine nuts, seeds and raisins and season with black pepper
- Combine with the herbs and rice, and fill each pepper
- Top the peppers with their lids and put them in a baking tin, with boiling water halfway up their sides to prevent them from burning or drying out.
- Pour 1 tablespoon of oil over them, cover with foil and bake for 30-40 minutes.

AVOCADO SALMON

The combination of the oily fish with the vitamin E in avocado makes this dish heart protective and a wonderful food for healthy skin.

200ml/7fl oz extra virgin olive oil
4 tablespoons white wine vinegar
6 tablespoons finely snipped chives
2 tablespoons coarsely chopped tarragon leaves
4 tablespoons coarsely chopped chervil
400g/14oz cooked, cold basmati rice
500g/18oz cold, poached salmon fillet
4 large tomatoes, roughly chopped
black pepper, freshly ground
2 avocado pears, peeled and sliced

- Mix the oil and vinegar with half the herbs and pour over the rice
- Flake the salmon, discarding any skin and tiny bones
- Add the salmon and tomatoes to the rice and stir
- Season generously with black pepper and stir again
- Sprinkle the rest of the herbs on top and serve on slices of avocado

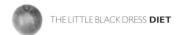
HERBY HERRINGS

So many people regard herrings as a food they eat only pickled, but try this traditional Scottish recipe and you'll soon be a convert. Great for dieters as they're satisfying, sustaining, and the oats add valuable special fibre which helps lower cholesterol and keeps you regular.

8 fresh herrings, split and trimmed

100g/4oz coarse oatmeal

black pepper, freshly ground

4 teaspoons caraway seeds

2 tablespoons finely chopped dill

2 tablespoons olive oil

2 lemons, quartered

- Wash and dry the herrings
- In a flat dish, mix the oatmeal, pepper, caraway seeds and dill
- Dip the herrings in the mixture, coating them all over
- Fry until golden brown, about 4 minutes on each side
- Serve with a wedge of lemon

SPAGHETTI A LA VONGOLE

This classic Italian dish uses small clams that have a very high brain- and energy-boosting zinc and selenium content. I find lots of people nervous about cooking shellfish, but nothing could be simpler than this recipe.

675g/1 1/2lb clams, rinsed thoroughly

225g/8oz spaghetti

55g/1 3/4oz unsalted butter

2 tablespoons extra virgin olive oil

1 small onion, finely chopped

2 cloves garlic, finely chopped

1/2 cup dry white wine

1 cup parsley, finely chopped

- Put the clams into a large saucepan and simmer in half a cup of water until they open
- Remove with a slotted spoon
- Strain the cooking liquid through muslin and reserve
- Cook pasta according to instructions on packet
- Meanwhile, sweat onion and garlic in butter and oil
- Add wine and reserved liquid and bring to boil for 5 minutes
- Add the clams, stir in parsley and pour over the pasta to serve

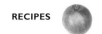

TOFU TREAT

Tofu is a basic food in the Far East, where obesity is rare, osteoporosis is virtually unknown and there is no word for the hot flushes which often accompany the menopause. Tofu is almost fat-free, rich in calcium and contains natural plant hormones which help regulate women's hormone systems.

200g/7oz tofu

25ml/1fl oz light soy sauce

25ml /1fl oz balsamic vinegar

2 tablespoons walnut oil

1 tablespoon crushed capers

1 tablespoon runny honey

4 tablespoons sunflower oil

1 pack of ready-prepared stir-fry vegetables

100g/4oz noodles, cooked

• Preheat the oven to 220°C/425°F/gas 7

• Cut the tofu into bite-sized cubes

• Mix together the next five ingredients and coat the tofu with half of the mixture

• Bake the tofu for 15 minutes, stirring occasionally

• Heat the oil in a pan and stir-fry the vegetables for 4 minutes

• Add the tofu and remaining sauce, turn down heat and warm through

• Serve with noodles

CHICKEN AND DATE RISOTTO

This delicious mixture of Middle Eastern and traditional Italian flavours is nourishing, sustaining and filling with the bonus of extra iron from the dates. Some people find that all the stirring necessary to cook a good risotto is too time-consuming; I love paying the constant attention that these dishes need and deserve. You'll find it absorbing and therapeutic – and think of the calories you'll burn.

225g/8oz thinly sliced chicken breast

1 medium onion, finely sliced

2 garlic cloves, finely chopped

1 tablespoon pumpkin seeds

350g/12oz brown rice

900ml/1½ pints vegetable stock

100g/4oz fresh dates, stoned and chopped

2 tablespoons parsley, finely chopped

1 tablespoon wheatgerm

3 tablespoons olive oil

• Fry the chicken in the olive oil until it's brown all over and remove with a slotted spoon

• Add the onion, garlic and pumpkin seeds and cook gently until soft

• Add the rice and cook for 5 minutes, stirring constantly

• Add the chicken, some of the stock and the dates

• Cook gently, still stirring, until the stock is absorbed. Continue adding a ladleful of stock at a time, stirring it in, until the consistency is firm but not too dry

• Add the wheatgerm and cook for another minute or two

• Sprinkle with the parsley and serve

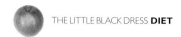

INDIAN MUSHROOMS AND PRAWNS

The immune boosting powers of mushrooms are legendary. Combined here with the zinc, selenium and protein in the prawns and the hot spices in the dahl, they boost the metabolism, as well as being highly nutritious.

4 large flat field mushrooms

I tablespoon olive oil

I large tin dahl, about 500g/18oz

I tablespoon sesame oil

2.5cm/1in piece ginger root, grated

225g/8oz shelled prawns

2 teaspoons soya sauce stirred into I tablespoon water

2 teaspoons fresh and chopped, or I teaspoon dried, chervil

I tablespoon each of chopped Brazil and pine nuts

I tablespoon toasted wheatgerm

• Brush the mushrooms with olive oil and cook under a medium grill for 5 minutes each side

• Gently heat the dahl

• Meanwhile, heat the sesame oil with the ginger in a wok or deep frying pan. When the oil is hot, add the prawns, soya sauce, chervil and chopped nuts

• Stir-fry briskly for 3 minutes

• Put a ladle of dahl in the centre of a plate, lay a mushroom flat on top and cover with the prawn mixture and sprinkle with the wheatgerm

PRAWN AND MUSHROOM BAKE

This is a perfect dish for anyone intolerant of gluten, wheat and other cereals as buckwheat is, in fact, a relative of rhubarb, not a cereal.

450g/1lb wholegrain buckwheat

2 large organic, free-range eggs

100g/4oz unsalted butter

2 medium onions, finely chopped

2 tablespoons extra virgin olive oil

225g/8oz thinly sliced mushrooms

250g/9oz prawns

I tablespoon chopped coriander leaves

400ml/14fl oz low-fat plain bio-yoghurt

3 teaspoons sunflower seeds

• Boil the buckwheat in 450ml/3/4 pint of boiling water until soft

• Beat the eggs in a large bowl and add the cooked buckwheat, stirring thoroughly

• Put the mixture in a non-stick pan and stir over a low heat until toasted and dry

• Use some of the butter to grease an ovenproof dish

• Put the buckwheat mixture in a dish with the rest of the butter and a pinch of salt

• Bake for 20 minutes at 180°C/350°F/gas 4. Check after 10 minutes and add more water if it looks too dry

• While the buckwheat is baking, sweat the onions in the oil until soft.

• Add the mushrooms and cook for another 5 minutes

• Add the prawns, coriander and pepper, stirring continuously

• When the buckwheat is cooked, stir in the prawn mixture

• Mix in the yoghurt, sprinkle with sunflower seeds and serve hot

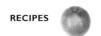

AROMATIC LAMB

*I buy all our meat from our fabulous local farm shop and
Karen, John and Alison, who own it, are always interested in how
their customers are going to cook whatever they buy there.
They looked a bit bemused when I said I was going to ROAST
the carrots with the lamb. But roasting carrots – even the big,
older ones you buy in winter – gives them a wonderfully sweet
flavour that goes brilliantly with this French modern classic dish.*

half a leg of lamb, about 1.5kg/3¹/₂lb

2 cloves garlic

4 medium sprigs rosemary

olive oil

1 large glass red wine

salt (preferably herbed) and pepper

4 medium carrots, preferably organic

• Trim most of the fat off the lamb

• Wash and pat dry

• Using a small knife, make eight cuts about 1cm/¹/₂cm deep
into the flesh

• Peel the cloves of garlic and cut into 4 slices each

• Wash the rosemary and cut each sprig into 2

• Insert a clove of garlic and half a rosemary sprig into each hole in
the lamb

• Gently drizzle with about 2 teaspoons of olive oil

• Season with pepper and salt

• Roast at 250°C/475°F/gas 9 for 10 minutes

• Meanwhile, top, tail and scrub the carrots – peel them, too, if they're
not organic

• Cut each of them into 4 pieces – once down the length, then each
piece in half across the width

• Reduce the oven heat to 200°C/400°F/gas 6

• After 5 minutes, add the carrots, baste the meat and vegetables well

• Continue roasting for about 1 hour, basting occasionally

• Remove the lamb and cover with foil, to let the juices set, for
10 minutes. Keep the carrots warm

• Put wine into the roasting tin and boil on the top of the cooker,
gathering up the crispy bits of meat left in the tin and adding a little
water if necessary

• Carve the lamb, serve with the wine and juices on top and the
carrots on the side

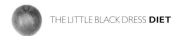

BEERY STEW

Could you get more Irish than this? Choose good organic beef to guarantee it's free from BSE, hormones and other nasty chemicals. The beef and the goodness of Guinness will together give you enough iron to make you magnetic, vitamin B12 for your blood, with a basketful of sustaining nutrients from all the vegetables.

450g/1lb lean stewing steak, cubed
4 tablespoons seasoned plain flour
3 tablespoons extra virgin olive oil
2 garlic cloves
450g/1lb mixed vegetables: onions, celery, carrots,
  broad beans, swede, parsnip, peeled, sliced and chopped
  into casserole cubes
300ml (10fl oz) strong beer or Guinness
Bouquet garni – buy the bags from a supermarket or make
  your own by tying together a bay leaf with a sprig each of
  marjoram, lemon balm and thyme
1 tablespoon lovage leaves, chopped

• Toss the meat in the flour
• Put the olive oil and garlic in a heat-proof casserole dish over a
moderate heat and soften them
• Brown the meat in the hot oil
• Add the vegetables and stir briskly for 2 minutes
• Pour in the beer and, if the meat is not almost covered, add
some water
• Add the bouquet garni and bring to the boil
• Cover and simmer slowly for 2 to 3 hours, adding more
water if necessary
• Stir in the lovage leaves just before serving

JUNIPER FISH

Juniper berries are a gentle, natural diuretic and their flavour goes perfectly with the sea bass. If nothing else, this dish will guarantee the elimination of some surplus fluid.

4 tablespoons finely chopped spring onions, including the
  softer green leaves
4 garlic cloves, crushed
2 tablespoons crushed juniper berries
4 tablespoons chopped parsley
4 glasses white wine
4 small sea bass – 1 per person
200g/7oz butter
olive oil
2 lemons, finely sliced

• Mix together the onions, garlic, herbs and wine
• Dot the fish with butter, brush with olive oil and put it in a large
baking dish
• Pour the wine and herb mixture over the fish
• Cover with sliced lemon
• Bake at 220°C/ 450°F/gas 7 for about 30 minutes, basting frequently

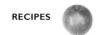

SPANISH RABBIT

I don't think Peter Rabbit ever reached Spain and Spaniards have no romantic illusions about Flopsy and Mopsy. Rabbit has less fat than any other meat – it's virtually fat-free. Combined here with prunes, for fibre and iron, and, with the stimulating benefits of horseradish, it makes a great entertaining dish when you're on the weight loss trail.

2 tablespoons olive oil
2 medium onions, chopped
1 rabbit, jointed and chopped
1 tablespoons wholewheat flour
150ml/5fl oz red wine
12 prunes, well-washed
1 large sprig tarragon
2 teaspoons freshly grated horseradish (if you haven't got fresh, a jar will do)
1 bay leaf
1 medium red cabbage
pinch of salt
black pepper freshly ground

• Heat the oil in an ovenproof casserole
• Fry the onions until soft, then remove with a slotted spoon
• Roll the rabbit joints in the flour and brown them in the hot oil, adding more oil if necessary
• Add the onions, wine, prunes, tarragon, horseradish and bay leaf
• Season, bring to the boil and simmer, covered, until the rabbit is tender - up to 1 hour
• Shred the cabbage, steam until tender and serve the rabbit and sauce on a bed of cooked red cabbage

VEGETABLE AND CHEESE CASSEROLE

Veggies will love this dish, but even dedicated meat eaters will enjoy the filling flavours of this vitamin – and mineral-rich, meat-free recipe.

1 green pepper
1 red pepper
1 yellow pepper
4 courgettes
4 tomatoes
olive oil
3 garlic cloves, chopped
3 teaspoons chopped parsley
small handful of torn basil leaves
2 tablespoons Parmesan cheese

• Wash and slice the peppers, courgettes and tomatoes
• Rub a deep casserole dish with olive oil
• Add the vegetables in alternate layers, sprinkling each with a little garlic, oil and herbs
• Cover with foil and bake at 180°C/350°F/gas 4 for 45 minutes
• Remove the foil, sprinkle with the Parmesan and return to the oven until the cheese is golden, about 10 minutes

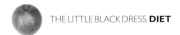

GRILLED SPICED CHICKEN

Allow one chicken breast per person and cook extra as it's delicious eaten cold the next day. You'll get extra calcium from the yoghurt, protein and B vitamins in the chicken and metabolic stimulus from the chilli, cumin and coriander.

1 large onion, chopped
2 garlic cloves, chopped
1 small carton natural bio-yoghurt
1 teaspoon coriander seeds
1 teaspoon cumin seeds
1/2 teaspoon chilli powder
4 chicken breasts, skinned

• Chop the onion and garlic and put into a bowl with the yoghurt
• Heat the coriander and cumin seeds for 2 minutes in a dry frying pan over medium heat, then crush them in a mortar and pestle
• Add the seeds and the chilli powder to the yoghurt mixture
• Flatten the chicken slightly
• Pour the yoghurt mixture over the chicken and leave the mixture to marinate for 1 hour
• Grill the chicken for 10 minutes each side, basting with the marinade, until the juices run clear. Serve immediately

STUFFED GRILLED TROUT

This recipe combines the health benefits of oily fish, with skin-nourishing betacarotene from spinach, plus some special nutrients essential for healthy eyes. The cleansing oils from the lemon make this a plateful of slimmers' nutrition.

4 trout
4 handfuls baby spinach
2 lemons, thinly sliced

• Gut the fish, clean thoroughly and pat dry
• Wash the baby spinach thoroughly – even if the package does say it's ready-washed
• Fill the fish with a layer of lemon, topped by the spinach
• Cook under a moderate grill for 15 minutes, turning carefully half way through, and serve immediately

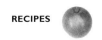

FISH PROVENCAL

This dish is suitable for hake, cod or any firm white-fleshed fish. The mixture of tomatoes and garlic is the traditional flavour of Provence. Both ingredients are good for the blood and tomatoes are full of lycopene, which protects the heart and helps prevent breast and prostate cancer. This dish is a true taste of France.

2 medium onions, finely chopped
2 garlic cloves, chopped
1 x 400g/14oz can good-quality chopped tomatoes
4 fish steaks

- Mix together the onions, garlic and tomatoes
- Cut squares of foil big enough to enclose generously the 4 portions of fish
- Put some of the tomato mixture in the centre of the foil squares
- Add the fish steaks and top with the remainder of the mixture
- Season with black pepper
- Fold up the parcels to make them airtight and bake at 200°C/400°F/gas 6 for 20 minutes

EASY LAMB STIR-FRY

You couldn't get a meat meal much lower in fat than this and, with the lamb, it's very filling and substantial. Stir-fried vegetables are quick to prepare and retain most of their nutrients. If you're in a rush, use a ready-prepared pack of stir-fry vegetables.

rapeseed oil
750g/1lb 10oz lamb fillet – or other lean cut, trimmed
   of fat and cut into bite-sized pieces
500g/18oz mixed vegetables, such as carrots or green
   beans, celery and other stir-fry vegetables, cut into
   batons
light soya sauce

- Pour a small amount of oil into a wok or deep frying pan and place over a high heat
- When steaming, stirring continuously, fry the meat for about 5 minutes, or until it is sealed
- Add the vegetables and continue cooking, still stirring continuously, for another 5 minutes until the vegetables are cooked
- Sprinkle over a little light soya sauce and serve

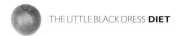
COD WITH YOGHURT CRUST

Coriander, cumin and paprika all help to stimulate blood circulation and the metabolism, making this low-fat fish dish ideal if you're watching your waistline. Nutmeg, by the way, is a mild hallucinogen and makes you feel good.

500g/18oz plain bio-yoghurt

1 onion, chopped

2 garlic cloves

3 tablespoons coriander seeds

2 teaspoons fresh mint

2 teaspoons ground cumin

2 teaspoons dried dill

2 teaspoons paprika

1 pinch nutmeg

2 teaspoons chopped parsley

4 cod fillets, about 175g/6oz each

• Put all the ingredients except the fish, into a blender and whizz for 1 minute

• Arrange the fish in a baking dish and pour over the sauce

• Cook under a hot grill until a crust forms and the fish is cooked through, about 10 minutes

PASTA AND TUNA FISH

Pasta is so versatile – and this dish couldn't be easier to prepare or more delicious to eat. It's just as good cold for a buffet meal as for a summer picnic.

500g/18oz short pasta – such as penne or pasta shells

8 plump spring onions, chopped, including the soft green tips

1 x 400g/14oz tin tuna, drained and lightly flaked

1 small handful chopped soft herbs, such as oregano, marjoram, basil, tarragon or parsley

• Cook the pasta according to the instructions on the packet

• Mix the onions and tuna

• Drain the pasta and stir in the tuna and onion mixture

• Turn into a bowl and scatter over the herbs

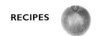

STEAMED SALMON WITH LEMON AND FENNEL

Even in the dead of winter, this delicate salmon dish conjures up memories of summers past – and those still to come. It's also incredibly healthy.

3 tablespoons capers
4 salmon fillets, about 250g/9oz each
8 fronds of fennel or dill
3 tablespoons olive oil
seasoning
1 lemon

• Drain the capers and soak them in some milk for 10 minutes to get rid of the saltiness
• Put some water into a steamer and bring it to the boil
• Put the salmon fillets onto a rack, place the dill or fennel on top, drizzle with 1 tablespoon of olive oil and season with black pepper and salt, preferably a herbal salt
• Steam the fish for about 8 minutes until the flesh looks opaque
• While the fish is cooking, juice the lemon, drain the capers and gently bruise them with the back of a wooden spoon
• Warm the lemon juice and capers with the remaining olive oil
• Remove the fish and serve, with the sauce poured on top

MUSHROOM RISOTTO

This delicious combination of crunchy Arborio rice and health-giving mushrooms is a quick, filling and nourishing meal. Serve it on its own hot with sliced tomatoes on top, or cold as part of a buffet or barbecue.

75g/3oz unsalted, preferably organic, butter
1 medium onion
1 garlic clove
50g /1³/₄oz mixed, preferably organic mushrooms
400g/14oz Arborio rice
about 1.5litres/2³/₄ pints vegetable stock
3 tablespoons chopped curly parsley, coriander or a
  mixture of both
4 tablespoons Parmesan cheese

• Melt two-thirds of the butter in a saucepan large enough to take the whole risotto
• Chop the onion and garlic finely and sweat gently in the butter for 5 minutes
• Wipe the mushrooms, slice and add to the onions and garlic. Cook for a further 5 minutes
• Add the rice and stir briskly to coat with butter. Add more butter if necessary
• Make sure the stock is hot and add 2 ladlefuls, stirring continuously until it's all absorbed
• Continue with the remaining stock, still stirring continuously, until the rice is tender. This should take about 20 minutes
• Grate the Parmesan cheese and stir in with the remainder of the butter and chopped parsley

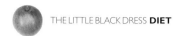

PUDDINGS

APPLE AND RICE PUDDING

Low in calories, high in energy, sustaining and delicious, this makes a perfect end to any supper – and, in fact, the leftovers are great for breakfast, too.

450g/1lb easy-cook white pudding rice
4 large dessert apples, peeled, cored and sliced
3 tablespoons runny honey

- Cook the rice according to the instructions on the packet
- Put the apples in a saucepan with just enough water to cover
- Bring to the boil, simmer very gently and stir into a purée
- Mix the apple purée with the cooked rice and add the honey
- Eat hot or cold

BAKED APPLE WITH ALMONDS

A feel-good fruity end to any meal. Nutmeg is mildly hallucinogenic, almonds are full of protein – and apples, of course, are the legendary way to avoid having to see the doctor.

4 cooking apples
125g/4¹/₂oz ground almonds
150ml/¹/₄ pint orange juice, preferably freshly squeezed
pinch of nutmeg

- Core the apples
- Cut off half of each core and put back into the core cavity
- Mix the almonds with the orange juice and use to stuff the apples
- Sprinkle with a little nutmeg
- Put into an ovenproof dish and cover with foil
- Bake at 180°C/350°F/gas 4 for 30 minutes
- Remove foil and bake for another 20 minutes until tender

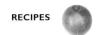

RHUBARB DELIGHT

This is a perfect dessert for slimmers because the rhubarb stimulates the digestive system and it's overflowing with protective anti-oxidants from the green tea. Enjoy it with a clear conscience.

750g/1lb 10oz rhubarb washed and cut into 2.5cm/1in
  pieces
zest of 1/2 an unwaxed lemon – rest of the 1/2 lemon coarsely
  chopped
2 tablespoons brown sugar
1.25 litres/2 1/4 pints green tea
1 handful fresh elderflowers, well washed (optional)
1 large carton of live natural yoghurt
8 mint leaves – 4 chopped, 4 left whole
1/4 teaspoon cinnamon

- Put the rhubarb, chopped lemon and sugar in a large saucepan and cover with green tea
- Place elderflowers in a piece of muslin, tied into a bag, and bury it into the rhubarb
- Cover, bring slowly to the boil and simmer very gently for 10 – 15 minutes until cooked, stirring occasionally
- Remove the bag of elderflowers
- Whisk together the yoghurt, chopped mint, cinnamon and lemon zest
- Serve the rhubarb covered with yoghurt and decorated with the remaining mint leaves

EASY COMPOTE

All fruit is healthy, but dried fruits contain highly concentrated nutrients which protect against heart and circulatory disease and many forms of cancer, as well as being the best ever cure for constipation – which will play havoc with any diet. Prunes have the highest anti-oxidant content of all fruit.

400g/14oz ready-to-eat prunes – Californian are best
400g/14oz no-need-to-soak apricots
2 lemons
2 oranges
3 tablespoons brandy
2 teaspoons sugar
fromage frais

- Chop the prunes and apricots
- Juice the lemons and oranges
- Mix together the juices, brandy and sugar
- Pour over the prunes and apricots and leave for at least 3 hours to let the flavours combine
- Serve with fromage frais

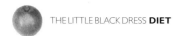

PINEAPPLE PUDDING

Anyone from Yorkshire might well be horrified, but this is Yorkshire pud with a difference. B vitamins from the wholemeal flour, healing enzymes from the pineapple, and immune boosts from the cloves, cinnamon and ginger make this a wonderful dessert.

I medium fresh pineapple, peeled, sliced and cut in chunks
4 cloves
60g/2oz soft brown sugar
1/2 teaspoon ground cinnamon
1/2 teaspoon ginger
175g/6oz wholemeal flour
60g/2oz white flour
90g/3 1/4oz soft brown sugar
2 free-range eggs
600ml/1 pint milk

• Layer the pineapple in a lightly greased ovenproof dish

• Add the cloves and the first lot of sugar

• Sprinkle with the cinnamon and ginger

• Mix the flours, the second lot of sugar, the eggs and milk and beat thoroughly into a batter

• Pour over the pineapple and cook in a preheated oven at 180°C/350°F/gas 4 for 1 hour or until set and nicely browned

CARROT CAKE

If you're on a diet you probably hate the thought of yet another handful of raw carrot sticks instead of the doughnut you're really craving. Here's the perfect compromise – all the healthy benefits of carrots in a light, crunchy, delicious, satisfying carrot cake. It's very nice and only the teeniest bit naughty.

2 free-range eggs
100g/4oz raw brown sugar
175g/6oz carrots, washed and coarsely grated
5 tablespoons light vegetable oil
100g/4oz wholemeal self-raising flour
1 teaspoon ground cinnamon
1/2 teaspoon ground nutmeg
50g/1 1/2oz raisins
50g/1 1/2oz chopped walnut pieces

• Heat the oven to 180°C/350°F/gas 4

• Beat the eggs and sugar together

• Add all the other ingredients and mix to a batter

• Spoon into a greased, lined 18cm/7in tin and bake until well-risen and brown on top – about 25minutes

• Test with a skewer – if it comes out clean, the cake is cooked

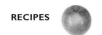

ENERGY BREAD

Offering a breadlike pudding to someone trying to lose weight must seem like giving a bunch of garlic to Dracula, but here's one you can eat. Thanks to the lime blossom tea, it's relaxing and calming. The dates give you lots of iron, so you won't get anaemic, and the betacarotene from the apricots is a treat for your skin.

5 lime blossom tea bags
225g/8oz pitted dried dates
225g/8oz dried apricots
200g/7oz soft brown sugar
1 egg, beaten
250g/9oz organic self-raising flour

• Soak the tea bags in 300ml/½ pint of boiling water. Leave until cold
• Squeeze tea bags into the liquid tea and discard them
• Thoroughly mix all ingredients and leave for at least 6 hours
• Line a 1.25 litre/2¼ pint loaf tin neatly with greaseproof paper
• Pour in the mixture and bake for 30 minutes at 180°C/350°F/gas 4
• Serve in slices topped with a dollop of low-fat natural bio-yoghurt mixed with a teaspoon of good apricot jam

TROPICAL HONEYED KEBAB

Nothing could be more simple than this exotic combination, and you'd never imagine that it could be part of any weight-loss plan. It gives you an enormous quantity of vitamins and healing enzymes, and the volatile oils from the sage are a powerful aid to digestion – essential for anyone watching the scales.

pineapple, mango and paw paw, peeled and cubed
a handful fresh sage leaves
½ teaspoon ground cinnamon
1 tablespoon honey
1 teaspoon lemon zest
1 small carton live natural yoghurt

• Thread the cubes of fruit and sage leaves alternately onto skewers
• Sprinkle with cinnamon, drizzle with honey and cook in a foil-lined pan under a hot grill till the honey starts to caramelise
• Stir the lemon zest into the yoghurt and serve with the hot spicy fruit piping hot

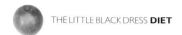

SPICY ENERGY CRUMBLE

A healthy variation of the childhood favourite apple crumble,
this dessert has lots of slow-release energy from the oats,
protein and minerals from the almonds, vitamins from the fruit
– and a fraction of the fat you'd get from a regular crumble.

450g/1lb mixed fruit (peeled and sliced apples or pears,
dried apricots, seedless raisins etc)
2.5cm/1in fresh grated ginger root
1/2 teaspoon cinnamon
6 mint leaves
2 teaspoon soft brown sugar
2 tablespoons water
125g/4 1/2oz ground almonds
125g/4 1/2oz oatflakes
3 tablespoons runny honey
2 tablespoons flaked almonds
60g/2oz unsalted organic butter, cut into small pieces

- Heat the oven to 200°C/400°F/gas 6
- Lightly grease a fairly deep pie dish
- Put in the fruit, ginger, cinnamon and mint
- Add the sugar and water
- Mix together the ground almonds and oatflakes and spread on top
of the fruit – you'll need enough to make a coating about
2.5cm/1in thick
- Dribble the honey over the top, sprinkle on the flaked almonds, dot
with the butter and bake for 20 minutes.

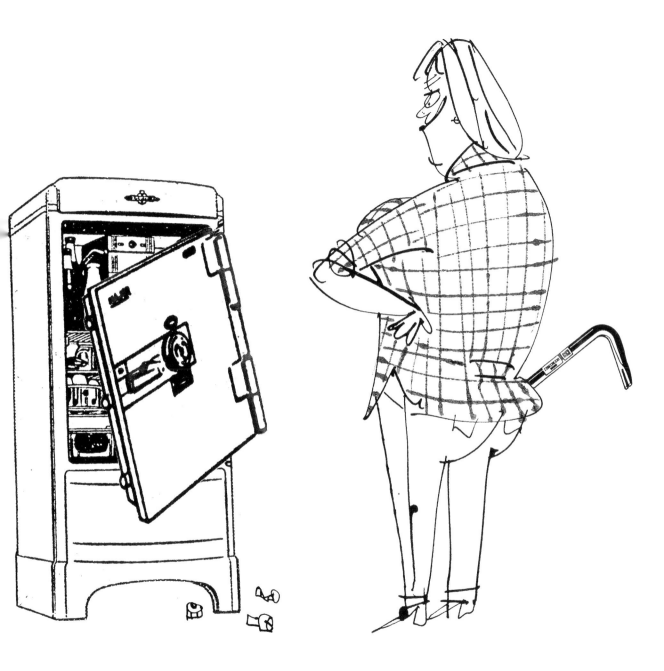

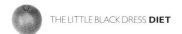
SALADS

This is the only country in the world where a salad means 3 leaves of limp lettuce, a tasteless overripe tomato, and 6 slices of see-through cucumber all doused in cheap vinegar, or revolting 'salad cream'. It does not have to be like this. Good salads are delicious combinations of vegetables, fruits, nuts, seeds, eggs, fish, shellfish, beans, rice, couscous and pasta, flavoured with fresh herbs, spiced with chillies, and tossed in delicate dressings. They can be a meal in themselves.

BREAD AND TOMATO SALAD

Nothing could be quicker, easier or more delicious than this typical Spanish salad. It's amazingly healthy too as it's rich in lycopene, which protects against prostate and breast cancer and heart disease, B vitamins and fibre and it contains cholesterol-lowering onions and garlic.

3 tablespoons extra virgin olive oil
2 cloves garlic, chopped
4 thick slices bread, cubed (crusts removed)
6 ripe plum tomatoes
1 sliced red onion
1 tablespoon fresh lemon juice
1 handful torn fresh basil leaves
black pepper
sea salt

- Heat the oil and add the garlic and bread
- Stir until the bread becomes crispy
- Remove with a slotted spoon and drain on kitchen paper
- Wash and roughly chop the tomatoes
- Put the bread into a bowl, add the tomatoes, onions, lemon juice, basil, and plenty of freshly milled black pepper and a pinch of coarse sea salt. Toss well

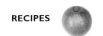

THREE-COLOUR COLESLAW

This attractive, crispy and unusual salad is delicious on its own served with crunchy bread, as a filling for a baked potato or as an accompaniment to cold meat or fish.

150g/5oz each of red, white and green cabbage

3 large carrots

2 crisp apples

2 medium onions

2 handfuls sultanas

1 medium pot natural bio-yoghurt

olive oil

cider vinegar

- Finely chop the cabbage
- Grate the carrots and apples
- Finely slice the onions
- Mix together with the sultanas and some natural bio-yoghurt
- Drizzle with a little olive oil and a tablespoon of cider vinegar

WINTER SALAD

This fruity dish gives a very unusual and sophisticated flavour to one of Britain's most undervalued but very nutritious vegetables. As well as being delicious on its own, it makes a perfect accompaniment to cold game.

1 large white cabbage – about 450g/1lb

8 ready-to-eat dried apricots

4 tablespoons shelled walnuts

400ml (14fl oz) freshly squeezed orange juice

1 small carton plain bio-yoghurt

4 teaspoons runny honey

the zest of 1 lemon

- Shred the cabbage finely
- Chop the apricots and walnuts and add half to the cabbage
- Pour over the orange juice
- Make a dressing of the yoghurt and honey
- Add to the cabbage mixture and stir well
- Grate the zest off the lemon and mix it into the salad, then scatter the remaining apricots and chopped walnuts over the top

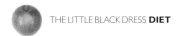

WARM SALAD OF MUSHROOMS AND RADICCHIO

This sophisticated mixture of radicchio, coriander and Parmesan cheese makes a wonderfully show-off starter or quick lunch. It would also go well with the mild flavour of grilled or poached white fish or cold chicken.

12 organic field mushrooms

3 tablespoons extra virgin olive oil

2 cloves finely chopped garlic

1 washed radicchio lettuce

6 sliced plum tomatoes

a generous pile of thin slivers of good organic Parmesan cheese

1 handful coarsely chopped coriander

black pepper

• Clean the mushrooms but don't wash them

• Heat the oil and add the garlic

• After 1 minute, add the mushrooms, cooking them on both sides for 3–4 minutes

• Layer 4 plates with the radicchio and a ring of thinly sliced tomatoes

• Put 3 mushrooms in the centre of each, pour over your favourite dressing – there are some ideas on pages 92-95 – and decorate with the slivers of Parmesan

• Before serving, sprinkle with coriander and black pepper

SUBSTANTIAL SALMON SALAD

Even those who don't like fish and would never dream of cooking it at home tend to enjoy tinned salmon. This simple dish, with eye appeal, makes a great starter or, in more substantial quantities, a perfect light lunch or supper.

100ml/3 1/2fl oz of your favourite dressing – there are some ideas on pp 92-95

3 tablespoons finely snipped chives

1 tablespoon coarsely chopped tarragon leaves

2 tablespoons coarsely chopped chervil

250g/9oz cooked and cooled Basmati rice

250g/9oz can best quality pink salmon

2 large tomatoes, roughly chopped

1 large red pepper, deseeded and thinly sliced

freshly ground black pepper

• Add the dressing and half the herbs to the rice

• Flake the salmon, discarding any skin

• Stir into the rice with the chopped tomatoes and red pepper

• Add a generous grinding of black pepper and stir again

• Sprinkle over remaining herbs

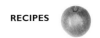

BEETROOT BOOSTER

Serve this creamy, pink mixture – based on a traditional eastern European combination of beetroot and horseradish – with crunchy, wholemeal bread. It's also a great accompaniment to cold meat or fish or anything on the barbecue.

700g/1¹/₂lb beetroot – cooked, preferably baby bulbs and
  certainly not pickled
the grated zest and juice of ¹/₂ lemon
I teaspoon fresh grated horseradish or 2 teaspoons
  ready-made
I heaped tablespoons finely snipped chives
I teaspoons finely chopped tarragon
I teaspoon finely chopped lemon balm
250g/9oz plain live yoghurt

• Cut the beetroot into chunks, or slice if large
• Sprinkle with lemon juice and stir in the zest
• Stir the horseradish and herbs into the yoghurt and pour over the beetroot
• Leave for I hour to allow flavours to combine

EGG AND BEAN FEAST

Here's a salad that makes a great main meal in 15 minutes. All the rest of the preparation can be done while the eggs are boiling.

4 eggs, preferably organic and free-range
200g/7oz can white cannellini beans
200g/7oz can red kidney beans
200g/7oz can borlotti beans
3 tomatoes
¹/₂ cucumber
6 spring onions
5 tablespoons of your favourite dressing – see pages 92-95
  for ideas
freshly ground black pepper
a pinch of sea salt
a small bunch of chopped parsley
a handful of torn basil leaves

• Put the eggs on to boil for 15 minutes
• While they're cooking, drain and rinse the beans thoroughly to remove the salt
• Roughly chop the tomatoes
• Peel and dice the cucumber
• Slice the spring onions lengthways.
• Put the beans, tomatoes and cucumber into a bowl
• Add the dressing and stir well
• Remove the eggs, run under cold water for 2 minutes, peel and quarter
• Put the eggs on top of the salad, cover with the spring onions then sprinkle with the herbs

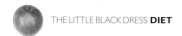
WATERCRESS SALAD

I ate this salad in a Chinese beach café overlooking the Indian Ocean in Mauritius, where watercress is the most popular salad vegetable. Okay, it might not seem quite as memorable on a rainy day in the UK, but it's delicious all the same – and perfect served with pasta.

I large bag or bunch of watercress
I large thinly sliced onion
the juice of ½ lemon
2 tablespoons extra virgin olive oil
a small handful fresh mint leaves
a small handful chopped parsley

• Wash the watercress thoroughly – even if you've bought a bag that says it's ready-washed, and remove any tough stems
• Slice the onion thinly
• Mix together the lemon juice and olive oil
• Then simply toss it all together.

CHICORY AND WATERCRESS SALAD

This was one of my dear late mother's favourite recipes – and every time I make it today, it brings back memories of Sunday afternoon tea. I make no apologies for including 3 salads based on watercress. It's one of the healthiest and most flavourful salad vegetables – and far too good to be relegated to a soggy garnish on a steak.

I large bag or bunch of watercress
3 heads of chicory
About 100-115ml (3½fl oz) of your favourite salad dressing – see pages 92-95 for ideas

• Wash the watercress thoroughly – even if you've bought a bag that says it's ready-washed, and discard tough stems
• Trim the chicory and cut into slices widthways
• Put the salad into a bowl and toss with the dressing

WATERCRESS, AVOCADO AND CELERY SALAD

3 large, ripe avocadoes
3 stems celery, with leaves
extra virgin olive oil
balsamic vinegar
2 large bunches or bags of watercress

• De-stone and peel the avocadoes
• Wash the celery, remove the leaves and chop the stems finely
• Put the celery stems and 2 of the avocadoes into a food processor and whizz quickly
• Add about 3 tablespoons of olive oil and 1 tablespoon of vinegar and whizz again until you have the consistency of a thick mayonnaise
• Slice the remaining avocado and put on the side of the serving plate with the reserved celery leaves
• Put the well-washed watercress in the middle
• Cover the watercress with the avocado dressing
• Season with coarsely ground black pepper

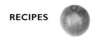

RAW VEG SALAD WITH BROWN RICE

Nobody can deny the health benefits of raw vegetables – and brown rice is bursting with good starch and fibre. This salad does take some time to prepare, but if you make extra, it keeps well, covered, in the fridge for up to two days, and you can use rice left over from a previous meal.

150g/5oz brown or mixed brown and wild rice
100g/5oz broccoli
1 large red pepper
6 spring onions
3 carrots
6 large radishes
3 large tomatoes
1/2 cucumber
5 tablespoons of your favourite dressing – pages 92-95

• Put the rice onto boil according to the instructions on the packet. Be patient – these rices can take up to 40 minutes to cook
• Either leave to cool or use rice left over from a previous dish but make sure it has been kept in the fridge
• Prepare the vegetables: cut the broccoli into small florets or half florets; cut the membranes out of the pepper and cut it into thin slices; peel and chop the spring onions; clean and coarsely grate the carrots; slice the radishes; chop the tomatoes; slice and dice the cucumber
• When the rice is cool – or warm if you've just cooked the rice – add the dressing and stir well
• Mix in the vegetables

PRAWN AND AVOCADO SALAD

Forget the tiny tasteless taken-from-the-freezer prawns smothered in pink goo and dumped into the middle of a browning avocado. This salad is light years away from that old cliché. It looks wonderful and tastes just delicious.

2 medium avocados
12 cooked Dublin Bay prawns
3 tablespoons chopped coriander
8 large tablespoons Green Dressing (page 95)

• Halve the avocados, remove the stones and peel
• Slice each half into 6 lengthways pieces
• Arrange the prawns and avocado slices alternately around the sides of 4 plates and sprinkle with the coriander
• Put 2 large spoonfuls of the dressing in the middle of each plate

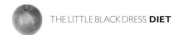

DRESSINGS

There's no need to spend loads of money on bottles of ready-made dressings – even those bearing famous people's names. It's far easier and cheaper to make your own – and you'll know that they're not full of stabilisers and other additives which are necessary to give them a long shelf-life. Making salad dressings can be time-consuming and messy but, if you like salads and eat them often, you can make a few days' worth in advance and keep them in a tightly-stoppered container. I use one of those beer bottles with a stopper like a kilner jar. You don't even need to whisk the ingredients – just chuck them in, close the jar and shake until it's well mixed. Keep it in a coolish place, but not in the fridge because the oil will solidify.

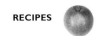

MY ONE AND ONLY

This is my basic dressing for any green salad.

2 spring onions
I clove garlic
200ml/7oz best extra virgin olive oil you can afford
200ml/7oz cider vinegar
I tablespoon runny honey
I tablespoon Dijon mustard
I sprig fresh rosemary
2 bay leaves
ground black pepper

• Chop the spring onions, including any of the green parts which are still succulent
• Finely chop the garlic
• Put all the ingredients, apart from the rosemary and bay leaves, into a jug – or pour into a bottle – and shake well
• Add the bay leaves and rosemary – and, ideally, leave to sit for at least a day to allow the flavours to infuse

MOREISH MOORISH DRESSING

This wonderfully piquant dressing is the perfect accompaniment to fish, poultry or roast beef.

I generous handful of herbs – parsley, thyme, chives and
  coriander
2 finely chopped cloves garlic
I x 450g/Ilb pot of low-fat live natural yoghurt
2 tablespoons strong horseradish sauce
2 tablespoons cider vinegar
I teaspoon paprika
freshly ground black pepper

• Chop the herbs finely
• Chop the garlic
• Mix all the ingredients together and whisk thoroughly

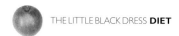

FIVE-FLAVOUR OIL AND VINEGAR

This is a dressing you'll have to say that you prepared earlier. It involves infusing herbs in oil and spices in vinegar for a week, but will give you a wonderfully individual dressing which is particularly good with sea food. So here goes . . .

250ml/9fl oz walnut oil

I sprig fennel

I sprig tarragon

I sprig dill

250ml/9fl oz best white wine vinegar you can find

I tablespoon coriander seeds

I tablespoon chopped hot, dried red chillies

- Put the walnut oil into a bottle and add the fennel, tarragon and dill
- Cork and keep in a cool dark place for at least a week
- Fill another bottle with the vinegar
- Add the coriander seeds and chillies
- Cork and keep them, too, in a cool dark place for a week
- To make the dressing, use 3 measures of oil to 1 of vinegar

DUAL PURPOSE FISHY DRESSING

Salads of warm green vegetables are popular around the Mediterranean but have never really caught on here. Use this dressing and you'll serve up a highly unusual health-giving salad which most of your friends will not have tasted before. The dressing goes equally well with salads of cold cooked pasta or use it as an instant sauce for hot pasta.

I x 100g/4oz can anchovy fillets

6 semi-sundried or sun-blushed tomatoes

2 cloves garlic

6 tablespoons extra virgin olive oil

I tablespoon balsamic vinegar

freshly ground black pepper

- Soak anchovy fillets in milk for 10 minutes to remove most of the salt. Dry on kitchen paper
- Cut tomatoes coarsely
- Peel the garlic cloves and flatten with a knife blade
- Put all the ingredients into a small food processor and whizz until smooth

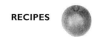

GREEN DRESSING

This dressing is perfect for tomato and onion salads, with cold duck or chicken, cold salmon or as a dip to serve with crudités of raw cauliflower, broccoli, carrot, red and green peppers, radishes, cucumber, celery and spring onions.

I handful watercress, washed, dried and chopped
I handful flat-leafed parsley, washed, dried and chopped
I tablespoon finely snipped chives
I teaspoon lemon juice
200ml/7fl oz low-fat mayonnaise

Put all the ingrdinets into a food processor and whizz for 20 seconds

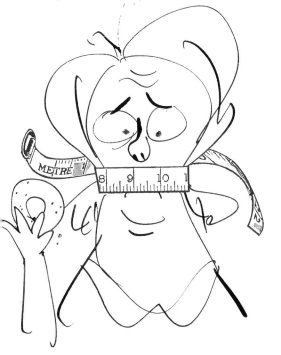

CREAMY FRUIT SALAD DRESSING

Instead of spoonfuls of artery-clogging double cream, use the light and surprising flavours of yoghurt enhanced with herbs and spices on all fresh or cooked fruits and fruit salads.

I x 400ml/14fl oz carton of live natural yoghurt
I whole unwaxed lemon
I tablespoon runny honey
1/2 teaspoon ground cinnamon
6 roughly torn fresh mint leaves

• Thoroughly mix the yoghurt, grated lemon zest, lemon juice, honey and cinnamon
• Stir in the mint

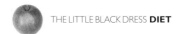

SOUPS

Soups are the perfect weight-watchers' food. Made at home, they're filling, sustaining and bursting with the extra nutrients you'll need when reducing your overall food intake. From thick enough for thespoon to stand up in to light delicious broths, they make a meal on their own or a perfect starter.

You can make soup out of practically anything – a glut of summer vegetables from the garden or the local pick-your-own, leftovers from Christmas lunch, the pile of salad and veg being sold off cheap in markets on Saturday afternoons or in supermarkets when they're still perfectly edible but they'll reach their sell-by date by the following day.

To my mind, making soup is one of the most enjoyable and creative ways of cooking. You can experiment with the produce you have or add herbs and spices to recipes you already know and arrive at soups which are truly your own ideas. Soups are so flexible, too. Serve them in attractive bowls and they're a brilliant first course for a dinner party, add crusty wholemeal bread and follow with some good cheese and they're an easy casual lunch. You can eat most of them hot or cold – and they're perfect poured into a small flask to give to the kids for their school lunch or to take to work; much more nutritious and warming in winter.

If you make your own, you know what's in them and you can freeze half to use later – which must give you a better and far less expensive nutritional choice than buying some commercial brands which are full of additives and cost a ridiculous amount for a can with two small servings. Remember, however, that yoghurt, cream, crème fraîche and other dairy produce should be added after the soup is removed from the freezer and reheated or allowed to thaw if you're serving it cold.

Making your own soup can be time-consuming, and it's tempting to take the easy option and use stock cubes as the base liquid. Not only are these expensive, they're often (but not always) full of salt and other stabilising agents, additives and preservatives. It really is easy to make your own.

Here's my recipe for a basic vegetable stock. On rainy Sundays, it's easy to cook a few litres, use some and keep the rest in the freezer.

BASIC STOCK

There's no need to fry the onions and garlic. All you need is water, vegetables, fresh herbs and a big pot. I always use a pasta pot with an inner strainer – all you have to do when the stock is done is remove the inner basket.

2 onions

2 cloves garlic

1 large carrot

1 leek

1/2 swede

1 parsnip

1 small turnip

2 celery sticks with leaves

2 litres/3 1/2 pints water

1 large bunch of mixed fresh parsley, rosemary, thyme and chervil

4 bay leaves

- Peel 1 onion – leaving the other 1 unpeeled as it gives colour to the stock
- Peel the garlic, but leave the cloves whole
- Wash, peel and trim all the vegetables (peeling isn't necessary if they're organic – all they need is scrubbing
- Slice or cube the vegetables roughly – it's not necessary to be that precise
- Put the water in the pot
- Tip in all the vegetables.
- Add plenty of black pepper, a pinch of sea salt and the herbs
- Bring to the boil, cover and simmer gently for at least 90 minutes
- Remove the pasta strainer or strain into a sieve
- Remove herbs
- Press all the vegetables through the pasta basket or sieve with a wooden spoon and add the purée to the stock

NOTE: You can add any vegetables which are in season, including green leafy ones. An easy way to store stock is to freeze it in ice cube trays then transfer to a freezer bag. If you then need small amounts of stock, you can just remove the cubes when necessary.

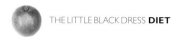
GARLICIOUS

*A traditional Spanish favourite, this fine aromatic soup is
bursting with goodness. It can be served hot or cold. In Spain,
the cold version often has peeled almonds and peeled white
grapes floating on top.*

2 large heads garlic
4 tablespoons extra virgin olive oil
800g/1³/₄lb young courgettes, trimmed but not peeled,
   cut into half lengthways and sliced
2 medium potatoes, peeled and finely diced
2 medium onions, finely chopped
1.25 litres/2¹/₄ pints homemade stock
fresh lemon balm, sage, rosemary and thyme, tied together

• Peel the garlic and roast it in 2 tablespoons of oil at 200°C/400°F/
gas 6 for 15 minutes
• Simmer the courgettes, potatoes and herbs in stock for 15 minutes
• Soften the onion in the rest of the oil
• Remove the herbs from the stock and continue cooking for
2 minutes
• Combine stock, vegetables and onions and liquidise

BEANFEAST WITH BARLEY

*This nutritious soup couldn't be simpler. It reheats well and a
large portion is filling enough to be a main meal. These
quantities make enough for 4-6 people.*

45g/1¹/₂oz pot barley
4 sliced carrots
1 chopped turnip
2 sliced leeks
2 celery sticks
1 chopped onion
15ml/¹/₂fl oz tomato purée
425g/15oz can kidney, butter, haricot or any other type
   of beans (except baked)

• Put 1 litre/1³/₄ pints of cold water into a large saucepan and add all
the ingredients except the beans
• Season with black pepper, bring to the boil and simmer for
45 minutes
• Rinse the beans thoroughly and add to the pan
• Simmer for another 5 minutes

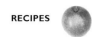

CHINESE STIR-FRY SURPRISE

Substantial enough to be a meal on its own, this soup has a wonderfully spicy Chinese flavour worthy of any top Oriental restaurant.

3 tablespoons sesame oil

1 red onion, chopped

2.5cm/1in ginger root, grated

1/2 dark green cabbage, shredded

2 thinly sliced leeks

2 sticks celery, washed and roughly chopped

1 large handful beansprouts

1 litre/1³/4 pints vegetable stock

1 large handful Chinese noodles

1 handful parsley, finely chopped

• Heat the oil in a wok or deep frying pan

• Add the onion and ginger

• Stir briskly until soft

• Add the cabbage, leeks and celery and stir over a high heat for 2 minutes

• Add the beansprouts, stock and noodles and simmer for 3 minutes

• Serve sprinkled with lots of parsley.

LETTUCE PRAY

Simple and delicious, this unusual soup has a real taste of summer, when lettuces are so plentiful. If you grow your own and are inundated with plants which all mature together, this is a great way to use them all.

1 medium onion, chopped

1/2 clove garlic, chopped

2 tablespoons olive oil

1.25 litres/2¹/4 pints chicken stock

6 lettuce hearts, thoroughly washed and shredded

225ml/8fl oz bio-yoghurt

1 handful fennel leaves

• Soften the onion and garlic in the oil

• Add the stock and bring it to the boil

• Stir in the lettuce and simmer gently for 10 minutes

• Add the yoghurt

• Serve hot or cold, sprinkled with the snipped fennel leaves

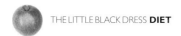
FRUITY, SPICY CARROT

Why we in Britain tend to disregard so many of our delicious vegetables, I'll never know. This quick and easy soup is very inexpensive, full of nutrients and looks spectacular served in white bowls as a dinner party starter.

4 tablespoons olive oil
1 large onion
2.5cm/1in fresh ginger root
900g/1¹/₂lb carrots
1.5 litres/2³/₄ pints water
500ml/18fl oz fresh orange juice
4 tablespoons single cream

• Heat the oil in a large pan
• Peel and chop the onion
• Peel and chop the ginger
• Sweat the onion and ginger gently in the oil
• Peel the carrots (if they're organic they'll only need scrubbing) and slice
• Add to the pan and stir to coat them with the oil
• Pour in the water and orange juice and simmer until the carrots are tender – 10-15 minutes, depending on how finely they're sliced
• Liquidise
• Pour into bowls and serve with swirls of cream on top

GREEN GOODNESS

The main ingredient in this soup is watercress, which contains not only large amounts of vitamins A and C, to keep your skin glowing while you're trying to lose weight, but also a natural chemical that specifically protects against lung cancer. If you're keeping hunger at bay with cigarettes this is the soup for you. It keeps in the fridge for a day or so – and is delicious cold with a small carton of cream, yoghurt or fromage frais stirred in.

1 large onion
2 cloves garlic
6 tablespoons olive oil
2 large bunches or bags of watercress
1.5 litres/2³/₄ pints vegetable stock
3 slices wholemeal bread, cut into cubes

• Peel and slice the onion and finely chop the garlic. Sweat them in half the oil
• Wash the watercress – even if you've bought bags which say they're ready-washed. Pick off any very tough stalks, but you don't have to remove all of them
• Add the watercress to the pan, turn down the heat and allow to wilt gently for 5 minutes
• Pour in the stock, bring to the boil, then simmer for 10 minutes
• Meanwhile, heat the rest of the oil in another pan and add the bread cubes, turning regularly until they're slightly crisp
• Liquidise the soup and serve with bread croûtons scattered on top

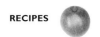

CURRIED PUMPKIN

*This typical American Thanksgiving Day soup is given extra
flavour and colour with the addition of curry powder. If
pumpkins aren't in season, use courgettes. Marrows are another
alternative, but as they're so watery add only half the quantity
of stock*

1 large onion
1 clove garlic
4 tablespoons olive oil
2 tablespoons curry powder
1 tablespoon flour
100g/4oz potatoes
1.5 litres/2³/₄ pints herb or vegetable stock
800g/1³/₄lb pumpkin
1 large carton fromage frais
1 large sprig curry plant or coriander or parsley

• Slice the onion
• Peel and chop the garlic
• Sweat onions and garlic gently in the oil until soft
• Add the curry powder and flour and continue cooking, stirring
constantly, for 2 minutes
• Peel and dice the potatoes
• Add to the pan with the stock and simmer for 10 minutes
• Peel and deseed the pumpkin and cut it into cubes
• Add to the pan and continue simmering until the potatoes and
pumpkin are cooked – about 10 minutes.
• Stir in the fromage frais
• Serve sprinkled with chopped herbs

GRASP THE NETTLE

*No, stinging nettles aren't simply those nasty little monsters
with a sting in the tale. This recipe uses the young tender leaves
to give a beautifully coloured soup with an amazingly delicate
flavour. You still have to wear gloves to pick them, though.*

100g/4oz young stinging nettle leaves, rocket, young
   dandelion leaves, sorrel – or a mixture of them all
50g/1¹/₂oz organic, unsalted butter
4 fat spring onions
3 tablespoons extra virgin olive oil
150g/5oz potatoes
About 1 litre/1³/₄ pints vegetable stock
Small carton low-fat live yoghurt

• Whizz the nettles or greenery in a food processor
• Soften the butter, mix in the leaves and put into the fridge
• Sweat the onions gently in the oil
• Peel and cube the potatoes and add them to the pan
• Cook gently for 2 minutes
• Add the stock and simmer for 15 minutes until the potatoes are
cooked
• Stir in the yoghurt and liquidise until smooth
• Return to a very gentle heat, add the leaf mixture and stir well

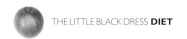
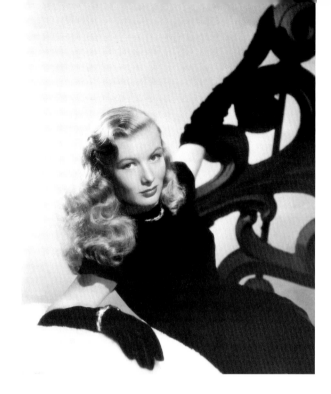

LIGHT MEALS, SNACKS AND STARTERS

TZATSIKI

Simple, low in calories and delicious, this delicate starter, snack or light meal couldn't be easier to prepare. Make a double portion and it will keep easily in the fridge for the next day.

1 medium cucumber
1 clove garlic
3 tablespoons olive oil
3 tablespoons chopped fresh mint
50ml/1 pint thick Greek organic yoghurt

• Peel the cucumber and remove the seeds
• Chop very finely
• Chop the garlic finely
• Stir all the ingredients in together and put into the fridge for at least an hour to allow the flavours to mingle
• Serve with pitta or ciabatta bread

MIGHTY HUMMUS

A Middle Eastern classic, this is an easy way to get good carbohydrates and lots of immune-boosting vegetables. Eat it with pitta bread and you'll keep the hunger pangs at bay for hours.

400g/14oz canned chickpeas
1 lemon
2 cloves garlic
2 tablespoons tahini
1 teaspoon cumin powder
125ml/¼ pint olive oil

about 50g/1½oz each peppers, cucumber, spring onions,
  carrots and broccoli florets

• Drain the chickpeas, but keep some of the liquid in case you need it later and rinse the chickpeas thoroughly
• Put the hummus ingredients except the olive oil into a food blender
• Whizz for a minute, then add the olive oil in a steady stream until it has the consistency of single cream. If it looks as if it's getting too thick, add some of the liquid from the can of chickpeas and whizz again
• Top, tail and deseed the peppers. Cut into strips.
• Peel the cucumber, remove the seeds and cut into baton-sized strips
• Trim the spring onions and slice into quarters
• Peel the carrots and cut into batons
• If the broccoli florets are large, quarter them
• Put the chickpea dip in a bowl on a large platter
• Arrange the vegetables around the sides of the platter and serve

Veronica Lake, 1944

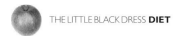

DIPPY DELIGHTS

These four dips are good with a selection of crudités including radishes, tomatoes, celery, florets of cauliflower, aubergine, strips of toasted wholemeal pitta bread or rice cakes.

SUPERAVO

2 large ripe avocados
1 clove garlic
1 teaspoon lime juice
1/2 red onion
1/2 teaspoon of chilli powder
2 teaspoons cider vinegar
2 tomatoes
a drizzle of extra virgin olive oil

• Peel, remove the stones and coarsely chop the avocado flesh
• Peel and chop the garlic
• Put the avocados, garlic, lime juice, onion, chilli powder and vinegar into a blender and whizz until smooth
• Turn into a bowl
• Roughly chop the tomatoes and drizzle with oil
• Stir tomatoes into the mixture and serve

OLD SMOKIES

2 fillets smoked trout
200g/7oz very low-fat cream cheese
1 tablespoon lemon juice
2 teaspoons horseradish sauce
1 small, fresh, green chilli
white pepper

• Remove the skin and any bones from the fish and cut the flesh into small pieces
• Deseed the chilli and chop it coarsely
• Put all the ingredients into a liquidiser and whizz briefly, leaving the mixture slightly lumpy
• Serve with lots of wholemeal toast

DIPPY RED YOGHURT

3 ripe plum tomatoes
300g/10oz thick Greek yoghurt
100g/4oz hot tomato salsa
1 tablespoon basil leaves
2 teaspoons lime juice

• Slice the tomatoes lengthways as thinly as possible
• Put the other 4 ingredients into a bowl and mix thoroughly
• Decorate them with the sliced tomato

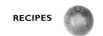

MINTY CHEESE

200g/7oz cottage cheese – NOT low-fat

100g/4oz natural, live, full-fat yoghurt

2 teaspoons extra virgin olive oil

1 teaspoon balsamic vinegar

4 spring onions

1 large bunch of fresh mint

• Whisk together the cheese, yoghurt, olive oil and balsamic vinegar

• Finely chop half of the mint leaves and stir them into the mixture

• Slice the spring onions as thinly as possible lengthways, including the succulent green bits

• Lay the onions on top of the mixture

• Sprinkle the rest of the mint leaves, whole, over the bowl

DIFFERENT DEVILS ON HORSEBACK

This recipe makes a great savoury dish at the end of a meal or in more generous portions a wonderful light supper.

400g/14oz organic chicken liver, cut into 4 thin slices

8 tablespoons olive oil

100g/4oz butter

8 small slices wholemeal toast

toasted pumpkin seeds

walnut oil

8 sun-dried tomatoes

thin shavings Parmesan cheese

• Pan-fry the chicken livers in the olive oil and butter for no more than 3 or 4 minutes, turning once halfway through

• Remove the livers onto kitchen towel and drain any excess oil

• Arrange them on the slices of wholemeal toast, cover with strips of sun-dried tomatoes, sprinkle with pumpkin seeds, drizzle with the walnut oil and cover with Parmesan shavings.

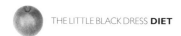

PRAWN AND MACKEREL KEDGEREE

3 eggs, preferably free-range and organic
100g/4oz cooked rice
225g/8oz watercress
175g/6oz shelled prawns
150g/5oz Cheddar cheese, grated
350g/12oz fresh mackerel fillets, skinned

• Beat the eggs and add them to the rice, together with the watercress, prawns and half the cheese
• Put half the mixture into an ovenproof dish
• Place fish on top
• Cover with the rest of mixture
• Scatter remaining cheese on top and cook at 200°C/400°F/gas 6 for 35 minutes

SIMPLE SALMON SUSHI

Seaweed is widely used in Japanese cooking and now available, with other Japanese ingredients, in supermarkets.

8 sheets nori (dried seaweed)
1 pack boil-in-the-bag brown rice, cooked and cooled
200g/7oz smoked salmon, cut in strips
2 peeled avocados, sliced lengthways
8 finely sliced spring onions
juice of 2 lemons
soy sauce
12 finely chopped Brazil nuts
lettuce leaves

• Cut the sheets of nori in half
• Put a tablespoon of rice in the middle
• Add a few strips of smoked salmon, a slice of avocado and some spring onion
• Drizzle with lemon juice and soy sauce, sprinkle with Brazil nuts, then roll the nori into a cone
• Serve the cones on a bed of lettuce leaves and enjoy with a glass of sake – Japanese rice wine, which is best served warm.

TRADITIONAL WELSH RAREBIT

300g/10oz grated Red Leicester or strong Cheddar cheese
freshly ground black pepper
4 tablespoons milk
a dash of Worcestershire sauce
a pinch of English mustard powder
a pinch of paprika
4 thick slices wholemeal bread

• Turn on the grill and line the grill pan with foil to save the washing up
• Put all the ingredients, except the bread, in a bowl and mash with a fork until it's the consistency of thick porridge
• Toast the bread on 1 side
• Spread the mixture on the untoasted side, leaving a gap round the outside
• Put under the grill until the cheese melts, bubbles and turns brown
• Serve with a salad of watercress, chopped onion and a sprinkle of chopped mint leaves, add a squeeze of lemon juice and a drizzle of olive oil

For a more substantial supper add a poached egg – they'll cook while the cheese is grilling. You can also turn this simple dish into a real feast by cooking 8 rashers of crispy grilled bacon – they'll cook on the grill pan at the same time – and adding 2 dessert apples, peeled, cored and each cut into 8 wedges, gently sautéed for no more than 2 minutes in a little melted butter.

BRUSCHETTA

This flexible Italian dish also makes delicious nibbles if you're having a party.

8 slices coarse wholemeal bread
4 cloves garlic
olive oil
6-8 tomatoes, depending on size

• Toast the bread
• Peel the garlic and cut the cloves in half
• Rub one side of the bread lightly with the cut side of a clove of garlic
• Drizzle with olive oil
• Top with slices of finely cut tomato

You could also add slices of mozzarella and put the bread back under the grill for a few minutes until the cheese starts to melt, or top the tomato with thin slices of avocado.

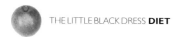

PRICKLY PEAR DIP

This unusual dish is great as a filling for jacket potatoes, as a dip for crudités or on a bed of cos lettuce with a mixed salad.

2 prickly pear fruit

1 avocado

1 teaspoon sesame seed oil

6 tablespoons extra virgin olive oil

6 tablespoons low-fat live yoghurt

- Scoop out the fruit and seeds from the fruit
- Blend together with all the other ingredients

WARM CHICKEN LIVER SALAD

400g/14oz chicken livers

2 tablespoons extra virgin olive oil

125g/4½oz unsalted butter

2 sprigs fresh rosemary

2 cloves garlic, crushed

2 handfuls watercress

2 large sliced tomatoes

2 teaspoons sesame seeds

4 tablespoons walnut oil

- Wash the livers and sauté in the olive oil, butter, rosemary and garlic until cooked through but still soft – 5–6 minutes
- Make a nest of the watercress in the middle of 4 plates
- Surround the watercress with tomato slices
- Put the chicken livers in the middle
- Sprinkle with sesame seeds and drizzle with walnut oil

GALLIC GLOBES

500ml/18fl oz white wine

6 cloves garlic

250g/9oz parsley

125g/4¹/₂oz chives

3 large plum tomatoes

125ml/¹/₄ pint extra virgin olive oil

2 x 400g/14oz cans of artichoke hearts

5 tablespoons torn basil leaves

• Boil the wine with the garlic for about 3 minutes

• Chop the parsley and chives and add them to the pan

• Add the tomatoes, oil and artichokes and simmer until the artichokes
are soft – about 15 minutes

• Just before serving, stir in the basil

• Serve with good coarse bread for mopping up the sauce

AVOCADO DELIGHT

Contrary to many people's opinion, avocados aren't fattening.

2 small wholemeal baguettes

2 cloves garlic

2 avocados

1 large bunch of parsley

4 tomatoes

2 small log-shaped goat's cheeses

4 basil leaves

**a few sprigs of fresh thyme – or a pinch of dried if you
can't find it**

• Slice the baguettes in half and toast the bread gently on both sides

• Cut the garlic cloves in 2 and rub the cut face on 1 side of each slice
of bread

• Mash the avocado just before you're ready to serve this dish so it is
a good fresh colour when you serve it

• Chop the parsley, mix it with the mashed avocado and spread the
mixture on the bread

• Slice the tomatoes and place on top.

• Slice the goat's cheese and lay it over the tomato

• Add a basil leaf for each slice of bread

• Sprinkle with thyme and grill for 1 minute

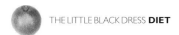
FLOWERY FISH

I really can't understand why most of us don't eat more mackerel. It's easily available, inexpensive, tastes delicious and it's full of heart-protecting fats, which are particularly beneficial for women as these special fish oils help with PMS and other menstrual problems. It's also, by the way, good to eat before a long flight as it will reduce the stickiness of the blood and make it less likely that you will get a deep vein thrombosis. In this recipe it's combined with lavender and beautifully peppery nasturtium flowers, which makes it a very attractive dish for summer – but is equally good when these summer herbs aren't around.

4 smoked mackerel fillets
250g/9oz cooked brown rice
4 tablespoons chopped coriander
2 tablespoons olive oil
6 teaspoons cider vinegar
8 nasturtium flowers
2 teaspoons lavender flowers

• This is so simple. Just mix together all the ingredients except the flowers – and decorate with the flowers when you're ready to eat

FISH FOR BRAINS / COLD SALMON FISHCAKES

All the oily fish are real brain food and this is an easy way to get youngsters to eat fish. These days, with so many overweight children and teenagers worrying about their diets, these are perfect for them and sensible nutrition for anyone else on a weight-loss plan. Eaten cold for breakfast, they're the perfect start to a high-protein day, which is why they're included in The Black Tie Diet. Here's my mother's favourite recipe.

1 x 418g/15oz tin red salmon
about 400g/14oz boiled potatoes
2 tablespoons olive oil
2 medium eggs
4 large spring onions
1 handful finely chopped parsley
6 tablespoons medium matzo meal
rapeseed oil for frying

• Drain the salmon, removing any skin. Mash well, including the bones
• Mash the potatoes coarsely with the olive oil. This is one time when it's okay to have lumpy mash as it adds to the texture
• When cool enough to handle, mix roughly with the salmon
• Make a well in the middle. Break in 1 of the eggs and mix again
• Finely chop the spring onions and parsley and stir into the mixture with 1 teaspoon of matzo meal and lots of black pepper
• Using your hands, shape the fish mixture into roughly palm-sized cakes. If the mixture is too runny, add a little more matzo meal
• Beat the remaining egg and put into a bowl. Put the rest of the matzo meal onto a plate. Dip each fishcake into the egg, then the matzo meal and shallow-fry in the rapeseed oil for 3-4 minutes each side until crisp and golden brown

MORE LIGHT MEAL IDEAS

• Watercress, avocado and celery salad with a chunk of
wholemeal bread
• A baked potato with 1 tablespoon of sour cream, fromage frais or
yoghurt and a generous sprinkling of fresh herbs
• A sandwich of wholemeal bread without butter, a mashed banana, a
couple of chopped dates, a squeeze of lemon juice and a sprinkling of
chopped nuts
• 2-3 large flat mushrooms or a good handful of button mushrooms,
fried in a little butter very gently in a covered pan for about 15
minutes and served on wholemeal toast with a salad.

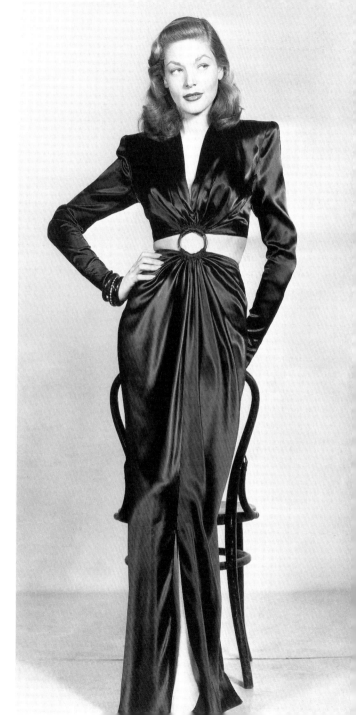

Lauren Bacall in To Have and Have Not, *1944*

INDEX